Audiology for the ENT Physician Assistant

by

Dr. Robinson Cummings

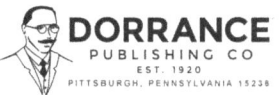

DORRANCE
PUBLISHING CO
EST. 1920
PITTSBURGH, PENNSYLVANIA 15238

The contents of this work, including, but not limited to, the accuracy of events, people, and places depicted; opinions expressed; permission to use previously published materials included; and any advice given or actions advocated are solely the responsibility of the author, who assumes all liability for said work and indemnifies the publisher against any claims stemming from publication of the work.

Dorrance Publishing Co
585 Alpha Drive
Suite 103
Pittsburgh, PA 15238
Visit our website at www.dorrancebookstore.com

ISBN: 978-1-4809-5096-2
eISBN: 978-1-4809-5073-3

Preface

First and upmost I want to thank Cristina Montejano, for her support in the making of this book. This will be the first book on this subject, and the idea was brought to my attention by Jose Mercado, MA, DFAAPA, PA-C. I have enjoyed what I think is quick and relevant reference to the new ENT Physician Assistant. I hope it's a useful reference in a busy ENT practice.

The primary purpose of the book is to provide a basic understanding of hearing disorders, characteristics of the hearing loss, and audiometric configurations related to disorders. The audiometric data is only part of the whole evaluation; however, it assists provider to select the subsequent appropriate test to obtain a diagnosis for the patient (i.e. MRI, CT and labs). In some cases, the etiology may never be known. With accurate audiometric interpretation the provider can often quantify the extent of the ear problem. Remember that the most important data you have is a thorough patient history of the hearing loss.

Chapter One
The Auditory System

The first thing you need to know about hearing disorders is the anatomy of the auditory system and physiology in order to medically evaluate the Hearing Disorder. The basis of learning any discipline is to start at the root of the subject you are trying to learn. Learning the basics allows you to rapidly pinpoint the source of the problem in the auditory system. The auditory system will be reviewed from the pinna to the brainstem. Sounds and speech travel from the source to the pinna as acoustic energy which is funneled by the pinna into the external ear canal to the tympanic membrane. The tympanic membrane converts the acoustic energy to mechanic energy which is transmitted to the ossicular chain to the oval window. The round window is connected to the inner ear which is connected to the Scala Vestibuli of the Cochlea. At this point the mechanical energy is converted to a hydroacoustic energy wave which stimulates the Basilar membrane which then stimulates the outer hair cells. The outer hair cells bend from the tectorial membrane movement converting the energy into bioelectrical energy, and that energy is transmitted to the inner hair cells which convert the energy to action potential which travels up the brainstem and stimulates the center of hearing in the brain.

Most common symptoms reported from patient are Tinnitus, hearing loss, vertigo and dizziness, otalgia, persistent ear fullness (after a flight/diving), abnormal sensitivity to sound (sounds seems too loud), wax impaction, decreased understanding speech in background noise, infection of ears, bleeding from the ear, chronic drainage from ear canal, trauma to the ear with hearing loss and/or dizziness, hearing their voice, loss of hearing acuity after taking medication or chemotherapy, baby failed newborn screening, and sudden hearing loss. As a clinical provider, your task is to learn and understand the types of Audiometric testing need to provide the patient with a reason and possible cure for their hearing disorder. Let's review causes of hearing loss and their audiometric data.

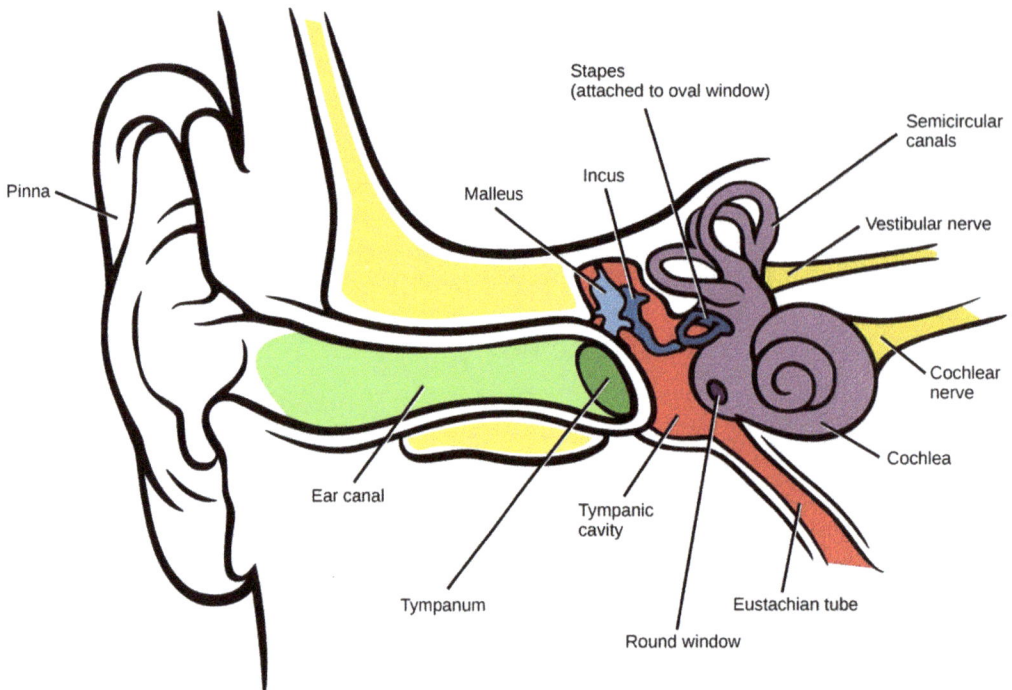

The Outer Ear

The outer ear consists of the pinna, external auditory canal, and the tympanic membrane. As noted, the pinna is structure to collect sound and channel the sound energy to the EAC.

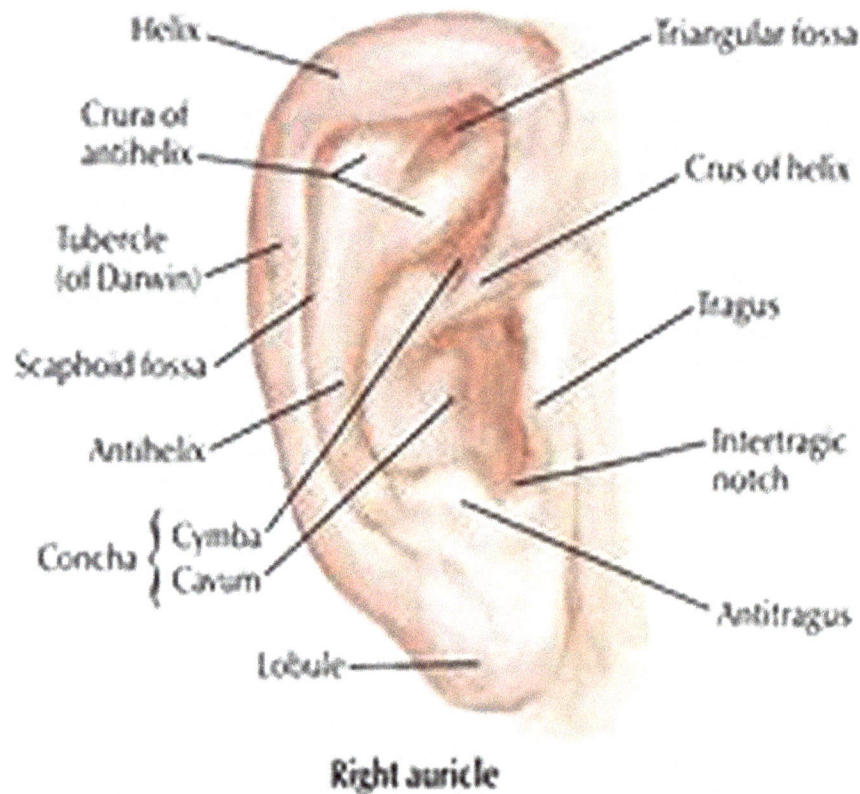

The canal allows the sound energy to travel through the canal to the TM. Some frequencies are allowed to travel through the canal with ease because of the canal resonance.

The ear canal is responsible for transmitting the sound and speech energy to the tympanic membrane. The size and shape of the external ear canal allow some frequencies past through the canal with less resistance which is known as canal resonance.

The middle ear has multiple functions which include converting the transmitted sound and speech energy to mechanical energy and transmitting the energy to the inner ear. The equalization of pressure from the outer ear to the middle ear is done via the Eustachian tube and mastoid cavity to allow maximum tympanic membrane mobility. The roof of the middle ear is a thin layer of bone separating the middle ear and the brain. Below the floor of the middle ear is the jugular bulb, and behind the anterior wall is the carotid artery. The labyrinth of the inner ear lies behind the medical wall, and the mastoid process is beyond the posterior wall. The space above the tympanic membrane is called the epitympanic recess. The middle ear is connected to the nasopharynx via the Eustachian tube. The lining of the middle and mastoid cavity is lined with the same membrane as the paranasal sinuses and Celia.

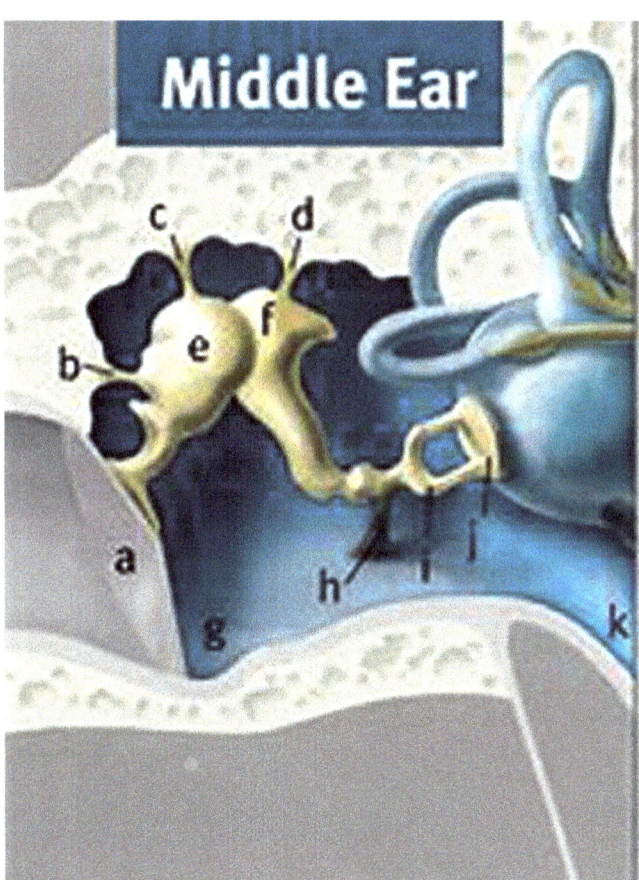

a) Eardrum

b) Lateral malleolar ligament

c) Upper malleolar ligament

d) Incudal ligament

e) Malleus

f) Incus

g) Middle ear

h) Stapedius muscle

i) Stapes

j) Stapes footplate and oval window

k) Eustachian tube

The inner ear is extremely complicated and is responsible for converting the mechanical energy from the middle ear to bioelectrical action potential to transmit to brainstem to brain. The inner ear is divided in two sections, one is the vestibular apparatus and the organ of hearing called the cochlea.

The vestibular organ is responsible for balance. The vestibule is two membranous sacs called the utricle and saccule. Both the utricle and the saccule are surrounded by perilymph and contain another fluid call the endolymph. From the utricle rise the three semicircular canals which also are membranous, containing endolymph and surrounded by perilymph. Each of the semicircular canals return to the utricle through enlarged areas called ampulla. Each ampulla contains an end organ called the crista which maintains equilibrium. The semicircular canals are arranged perpendicular to the ear other so as to cover all dimension of space. With any acceleration or movement of the head, at least one semicircular canal is stimulated which allows the individual to know where he is at all times in space and when he or a vehicle is moving or stopping. This process is complicated; however, this is basic explanation of function and when any portion of the balance is working correctly the patient has vertigo.

The cochlea is responsible for hearing. The organ has the spectrum of hearing frequencies for a human which is 20 Hz to 20,000 Hz. The 20,000 Hz is located at the base of the cochlea to the top of the cochlea which is 20 Hz. It houses the organ or cot which resides in the Basilar membrane one of the three walls of the Scalia media. Situated on the basilar membrane are three of five parallel rows of 12,000 to 15,000 outer hair cells and one row of 3,000 inner hair cells where the auditory nerve connects. These hair cells are stimulated when the sound energy is introduced via the round window stimulating the Reissner's membrane where the sound wave occurs as a stimulation of the staples from the middle ear. This wave-like movement of the endolymph stimulates the basilar membrane from the base to the apex of the cochlea. The tectorial membrane then stimulates the inner hair cells which convert the action potential to the outer hair cell to transmit the message to the brain via the auditory portion of the eight nerves.

A Word about Hair Cells

- Hair Cells are the reason that we can detect and understand sounds.
- The hair cells are set up "tonotopically" in the cochlea. Our range of hearing is from 20 Hz to 20,000 HZ.

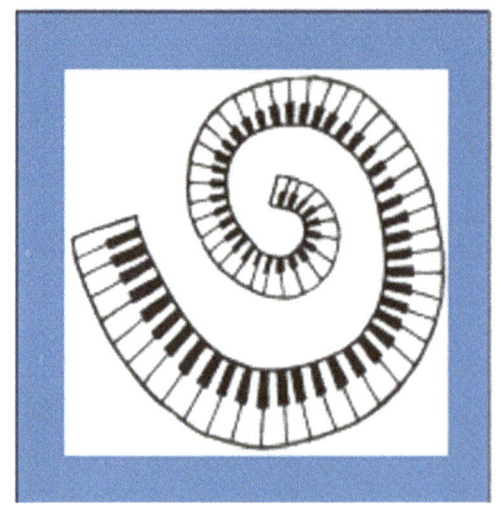

Cross sectional view of Cochlea

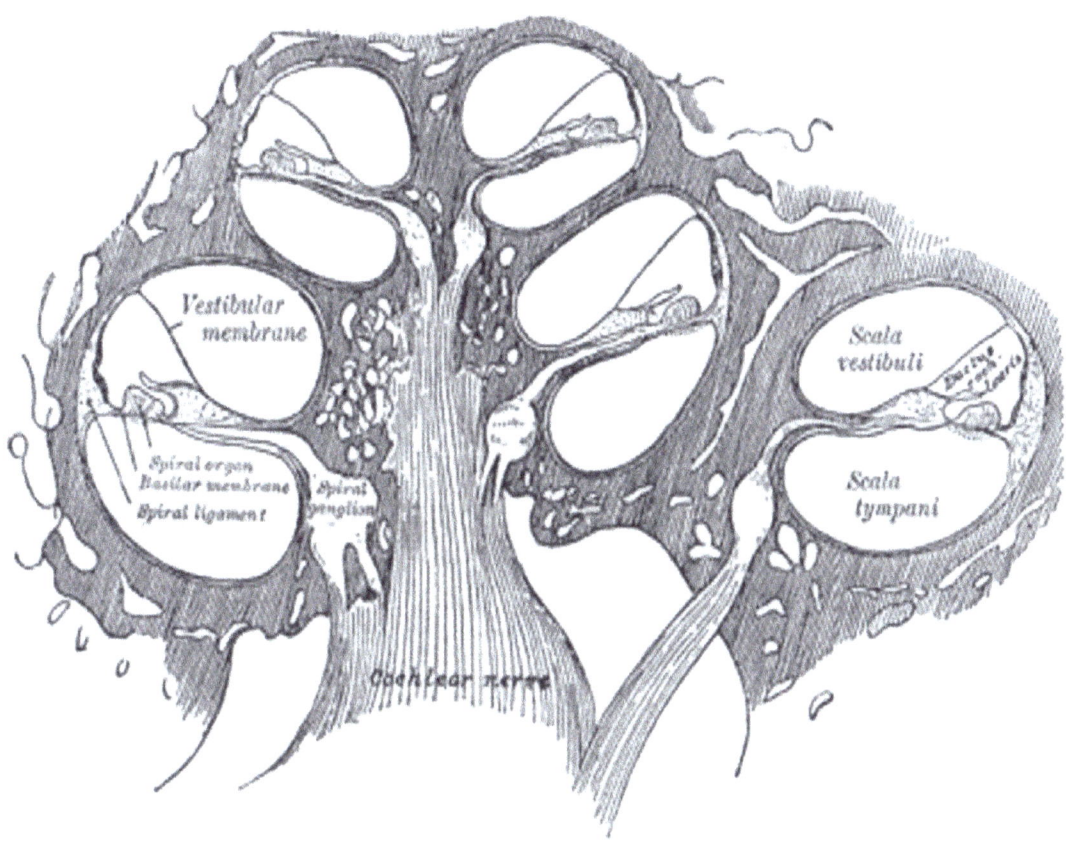

Below is an electron microscope photograph of normal hair cells. Very organized.

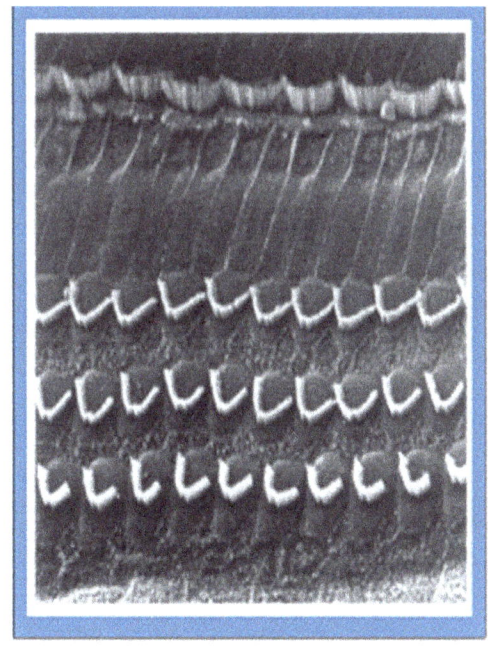

The Impaired Ear

This is an electron microscope photograph of damaged hair cells. When hair cells are damaged, they cannot be repaired or replaced.

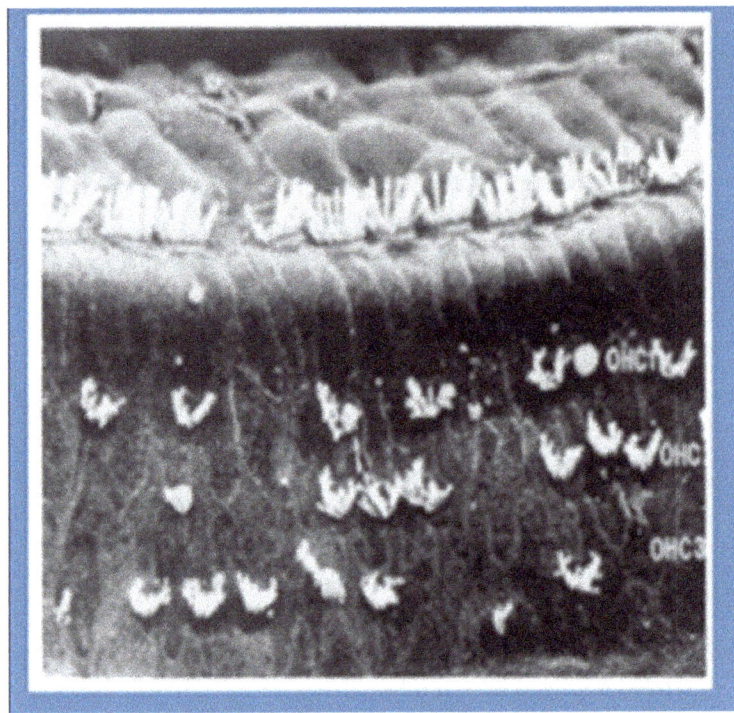

The diagram provided below is a graph presentation of the 8th nerve as it tracks up the brain stem to the Auditory Cortex. An important site to on the first synapse on the Ventral Cochlear Nucleus is where the facial branch of the facial nerve synapses, which are important for the blink reflex which is absent in the case of large acoustic neuroma.

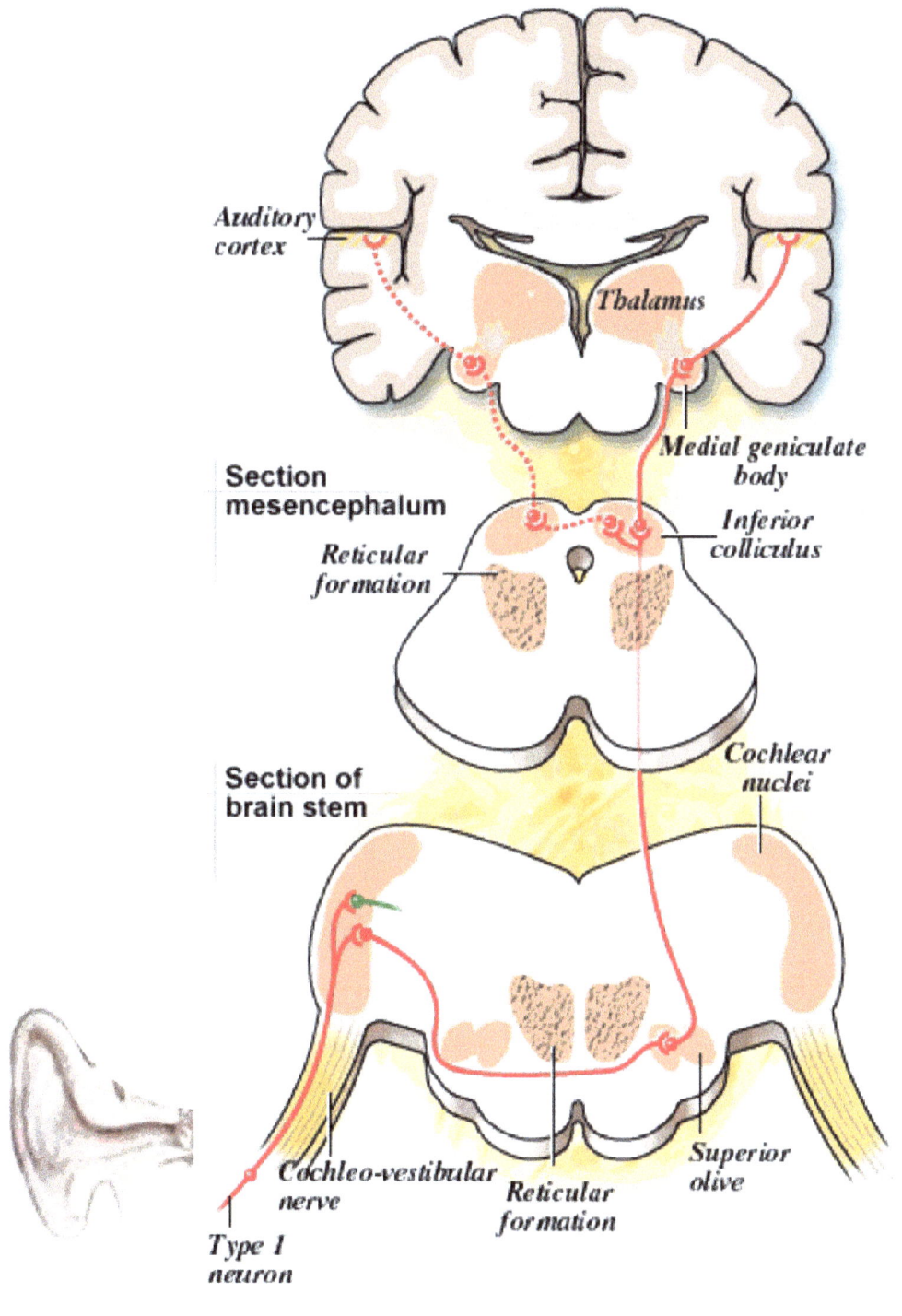

The Infant Ear

The anatomy of the infant ear is different from the adult ear. Size of the outer ear, middle ear, and mastoid. Mass changes of the middle ear are due to bone density and mesenchyme (a loosely organized mainly mesodermal embryonic tissue that develops into connective and skeletal tissue), change of the membrane system, formation of bony ear canal wall, and changes in ossicular joint. The infant ear is mass-dominated. The infant ear has a lower resonance frequency; therefore, lower probe tones create complex patterns and more notching. Classification scheme not consistent with pathology for example the infant has effusion and you receive a Type A tympanogram. With infants, you have to test with a 1000Hz probe tone is optimal.

Chapter Two

Audiometric Testing

Pure tone audiometric is performed to determine the softest decibel threshold at which the patient can hear the sound 50% of the time in each frequency from 250 Hz to 8,000 Hz or all test frequencies. The determined pure tone thresholds are plotted on the audiogram graph showing hearing threshold (dB) as a function of frequency (Hz). The audiogram graph is laid out in the format of frequencies across the top 250 to 8,000 Hz on the horizontal plane and the vertical place the loudness is labeled from -10 to 120 dBs' Normal hearing thresholds for all test frequency are from -10 to 20 dB HL, mild hearing loss is from 20 to 40 dB HL, moderate hearing loss is from 40 to 60 dB HL, severe hearing loss is from 60 to 80 dB HL, and profound hearing loss is greater than 80 dB HL.

Audiological Test Battery

Comprehensive Audiometric Testing: Evaluates the overall acuity of the hearing system from the tympanic membrane to the cortex of the brain.

Tympanogram: Evaluates the function of the Tympanic Membrane and Ossicular Chain and Middle Ear Space.

Otoacoustic Emissions: Evaluates the Gutter Hair Cells of the Cochlea.

Evoked Potentials Testing:
  a. Auditory Brainstem Response: Evaluate the 8th nerve from the cochlea to the cerebral cortex to determine site of lesion.
  b. Electrocochleargram: Evaluate the cochlea for increase endolymphatic fluid. Use to evaluate for Ménières.
  c. Vestibular Evoked Myogenic Potential: Evaluates the Otolith of the saccule and utricle (Upper and lower branch of the eighth nerve) which is used to evaluate for Superior Canal Dehiscence.

Vestibular Nystagmogram (VNG): Evaluates the vestibular system for lesions that are Central of Peripheral.

Video Head Impulse Testing (vHit): evaluates all Semicircular Canals. Semicircular Canal specific testing.

Rotary Chair Testing: Evaluates the vestibular system for bilateral weakness.

Posturography Testing: evaluates the 3 major causes of dizziness, Visual, Vestibular and Somatosensory lesions.

Speech & the Audiogram Example

- This patient has normal hearing in the low frequencies and will have no trouble with low frequency speech sounds.
- Sloping loss in the higher frequencies will make it difficult to hear consonant sounds such as "k", "f", "s", and "th" at a normal conversation level.

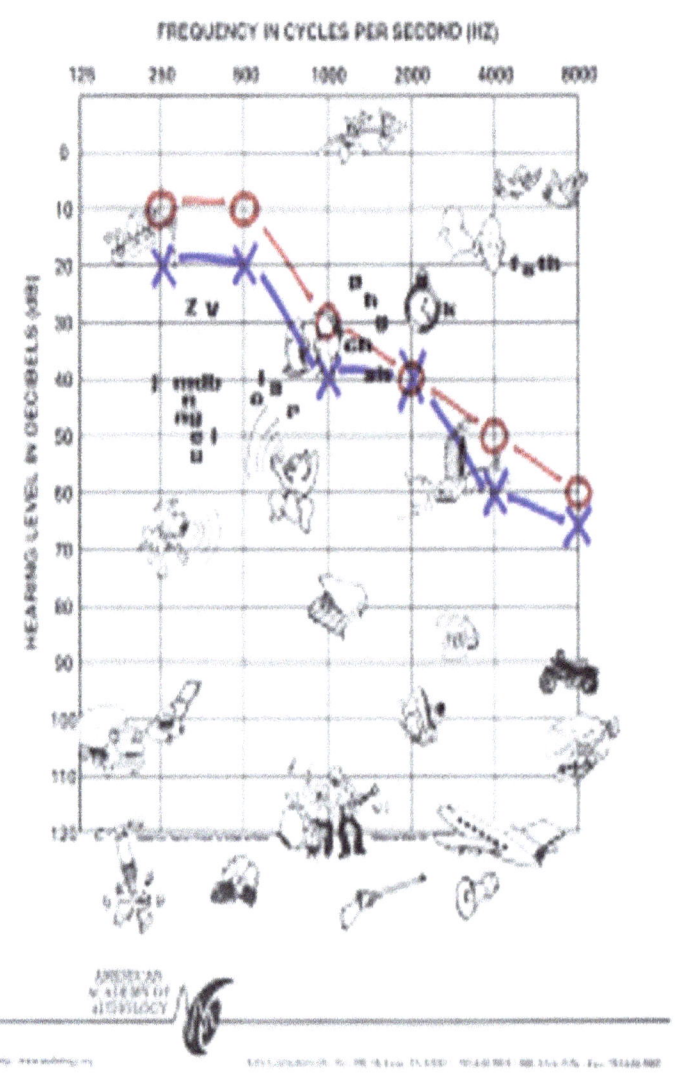

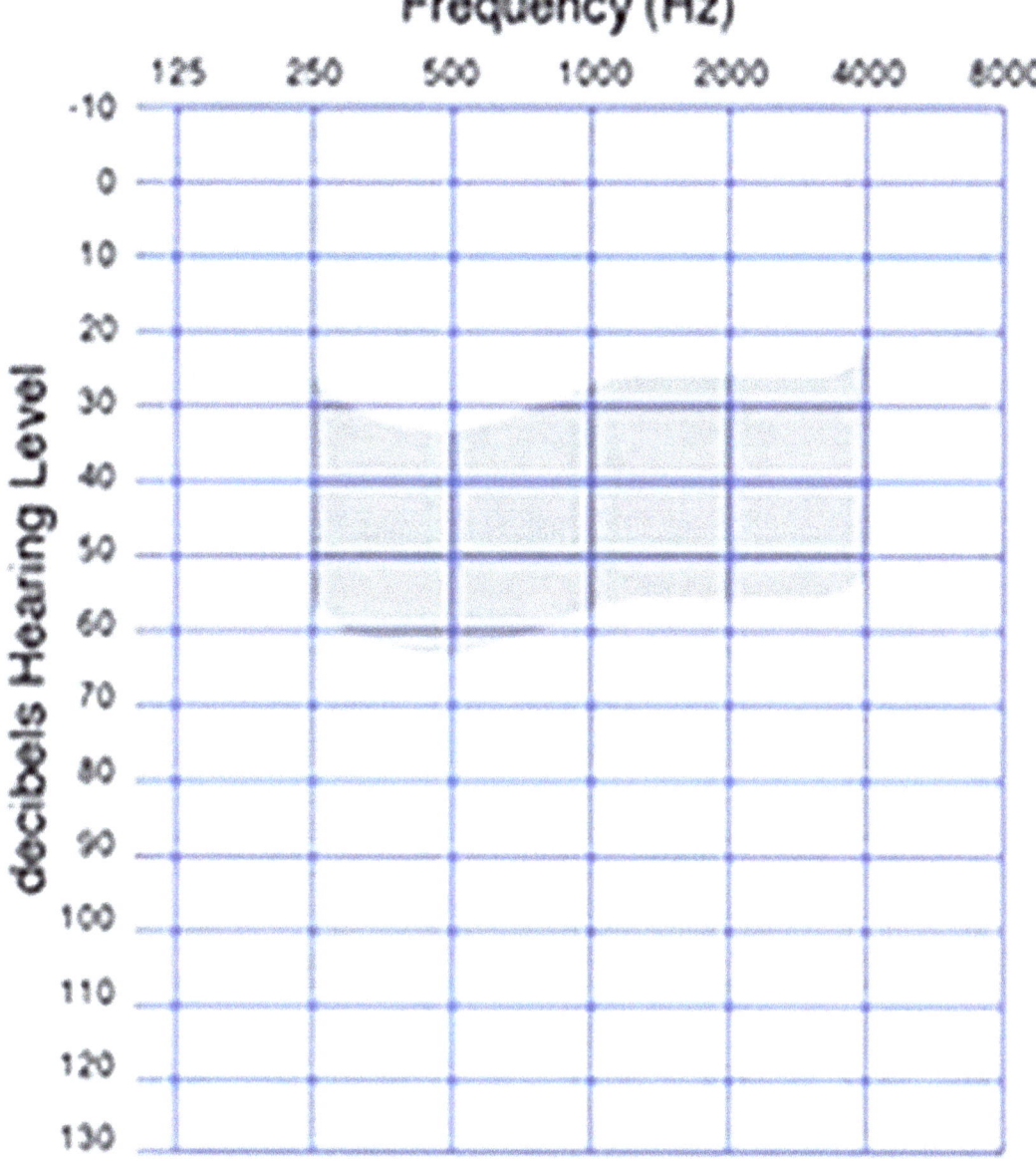

Speech Audiometry

Speech Audiometry consists of two parts: the speech reception threshold and word discrimination score. The speech reception threshold is the softest level at which the patient can correctly repeat 50% of the presented spondee words. Spondee words are two syllable words such as cowboy, airplane, and sidewalk, where both parts of the word have equal energy. The speech reception threshold is recorded in decibels and serves as a crosscheck for the pure tone air conductions threshold. The speech discrimination score is the percentage of correct phonetically balanced words obtains from the test patient when presented at his comfort speech level of speech understanding. Phonetically balanced words are the most common words use in a normal conversation. The speech discrimination score has two purposes. The first is to establish the prognosis for the use of a hearing aid and to determine the site of lesion. A poor discrimination score usually indicates significant neural degeneration which makes the prognosis of using hearing aid poor and then the clinician can look at Cochlear implant recommendation. Poor discrimination with normal or near normal pure tone thresholds is indicative of a central lesion.

Visual Reinforcement Audiometry

Visual reinforcement audiometry—Visual reinforcement audiometry (VRA) is used to evaluate the hearing of infants and young children from about six months of age through the second year. Sound stimuli (live voice and tones) are presented in the sound field and via inserted earphones. The child is visually rewarded with lighted and animated toys for turning his or her head toward the sound source. The child is conditioned to perform this task repeatedly. An experienced audiologist will use several lighted and animated toys and an intermittent reinforcement schedule to maintain the child's attention. Under ideal circumstances, complete ear-specific information for speech stimuli and interactive frequencies from 250 through 8000 Hz can be obtained.

Behavioral Observation Audiometry

Behavioral observation audiometry (BOA) is used to examine auditory function in infants younger than six to eight months, children with multiple handicaps, or adults who are not able to cooperate for other types of testing. Live voice, warbled tones, or narrow-band noises are presented in a sound field environment to elicit reflexive and orienting responses to auditory stimuli. The responses can include head or limb reflex, whole-body startle, sucking, eye blinking, raising of the eyebrows, or cessation of certain behaviors, such as movement or sucking. Responses to stimuli are not reinforced.

Evaluation of Hearing Loss, Weber and Rinne Tests

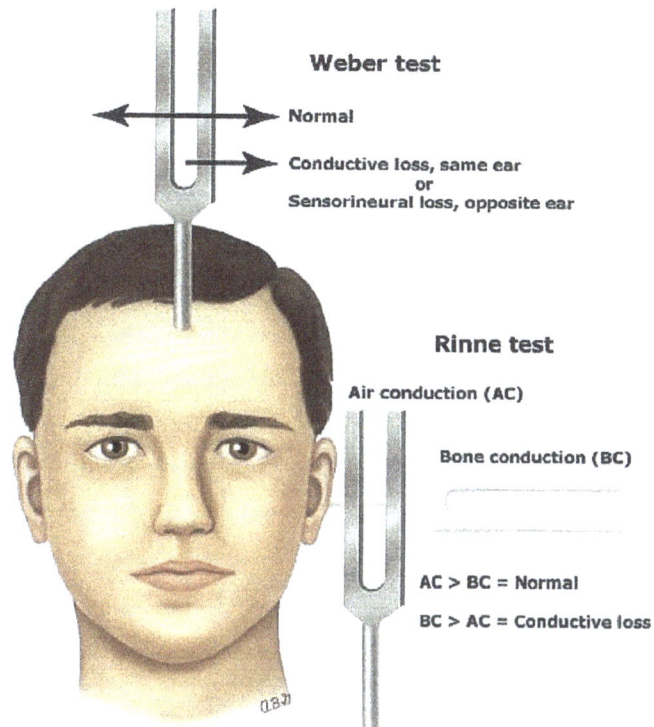

Weber Test: Place the base of a struck tuning fork on the bridge of the forehead, nose, or teeth. In a normal test, there is no lateralization of sound. With unilateral conductive loss, sound lateralizes towards affected ear. With unilateral sensorineural loss, sound lateralizes to the normal or better-hearing side.

Rinne Test: Place the base of a struck tuning fork on the mastoid bone behind the ear. Have the patient indicate when sound is no longer heard. Move fork (held at base) beside ear and ask if now audible. In a normal test, AC > BC; patient can hear fork at ear. With conductive loss, BC > AC; patient will not hear fork at ear.

AC: air conduction; BC: bone conduction.

Summary of test results in normal, conductive, and sensorineural hearing loss

	Weber test lateralizes	Rinne test	Pure tone audiometry		Tympanometry	ABR
			Air	Bone		
Normal hearing	No	Positive	Normal (0 to 20 dB)	Normal (0 to 20 dB)	Type A	Normal
Conductive hearing loss						
Good ear	No	Positive	Normal	Normal	Type A	Normal
Bad ear	Yes	Negative	Abnormal (>20 dB)	Normal	Type B, C, AS, or AD	
Sensorineural hearing loss						
Good ear	Yes	Positive	Normal	Normal	Type A	Normal
Bad ear	No	Positive	Abnormal (>20 dB)	Abnormal (>20 dB)	Type A	Abnormal (delayed or absent waves)

ABR: auditory brainstem response; dB: decibels; AS: type A tympanogram with reduced compliance (shallow); AD: type A tympanogram with increased compliance (deep).

Tympanometry

Tympanometry is an examination used to test the condition of the outer, middle ear, and mobility of the tympanic membrane and the conduction bones by creating variations of air pressure in the ear canal.

Tympanometry is an objective test of middle-ear function. It's a measure of energy transmission through the outer and middle ear. The test should not be used to assess the sensitivity of hearing and the results of this test should always be viewed in conjunction with pure tone audiometry. Tympanometry is a valuable component of the audiometric evaluation. In evaluating hearing loss, tympanometry permits a distinction between sensorineural and conductive hearing loss, when evaluation is not apparent via Weber and Rinne testing. Tympanometry can be helpful in making the diagnosis of otitis media by demonstrating the presence of a middle ear effusion or cholesteatoma.

Tympanometry

A tone of 226 Hz is generated by the tympanometer into the ear canal, where the sound strikes the tympanic membrane, causing vibration of the middle ear, which in turn results in the conscious perception of hearing. Some of this sound is reflected back and picked up by the instrument. Most middle ear problems result in stiffening of the middle ear, which causes more of the sound to be reflected back.

Admittance is how energy is transmitted through the middle ear. The instrument measures the reflected sound and expresses it as an admittance or compliance, plotting the results on a chart known as a tympanogram.

Normally, the air pressure in the ear canal is the same as ambient pressure. Also, under normal conditions, the air pressure in the middle ear is approximately the same as ambient pressure since the Eustachian tube opens periodically to ventilate the middle ear and to equalize pressure. In a healthy individual, the maximum sound is transmitted through the middle ear when the ambient air pressure in the ear canal is equal to the pressure in the middle ear.

After an otoscopy (examination of the ear with an otoscope) to ensure that the path to the eardrum is clear and that there is no perforation, the test is performed by inserting the tympanometer probe in the ear canal. The instrument changes the pressure in the ear, generates a pure tone, and measures the eardrum responses to the sound at different pressures. This produces a series of data measuring how admittance varies with pressure, which is plotted as a tympanogram.

One method of classifying tympanograms:

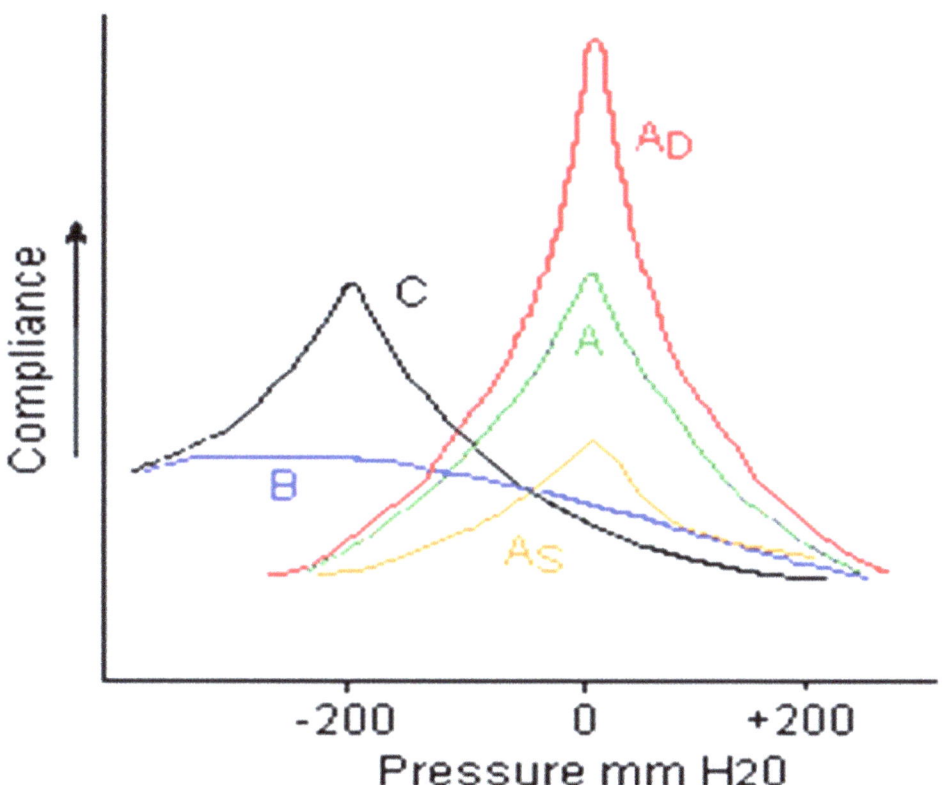

Indication of tympanometry graph

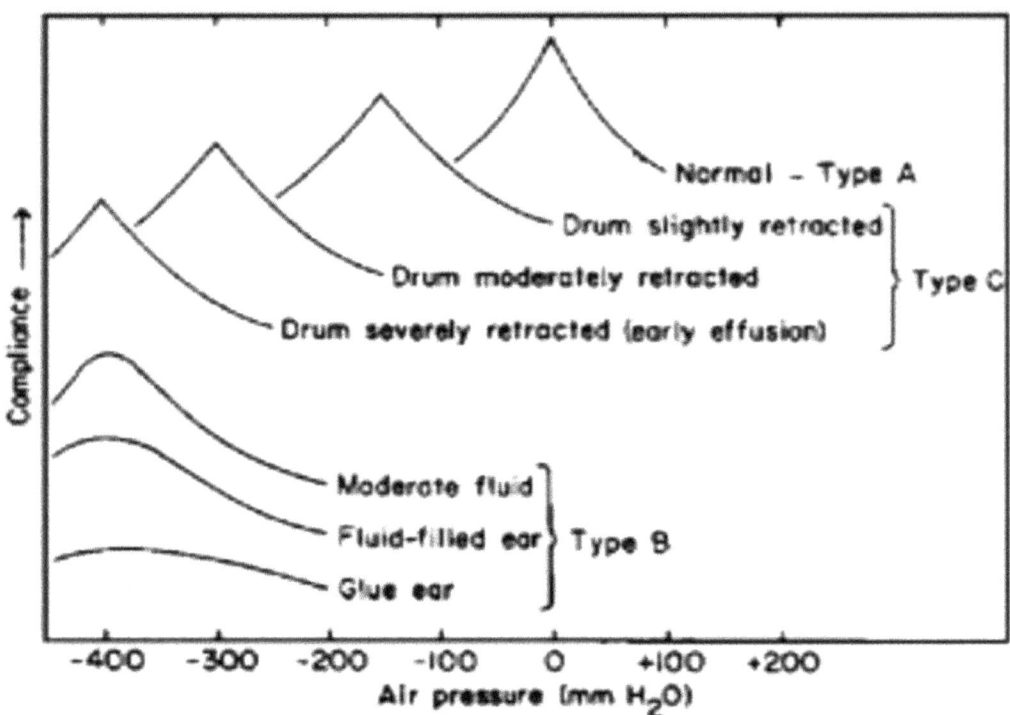

Type A tympanogram

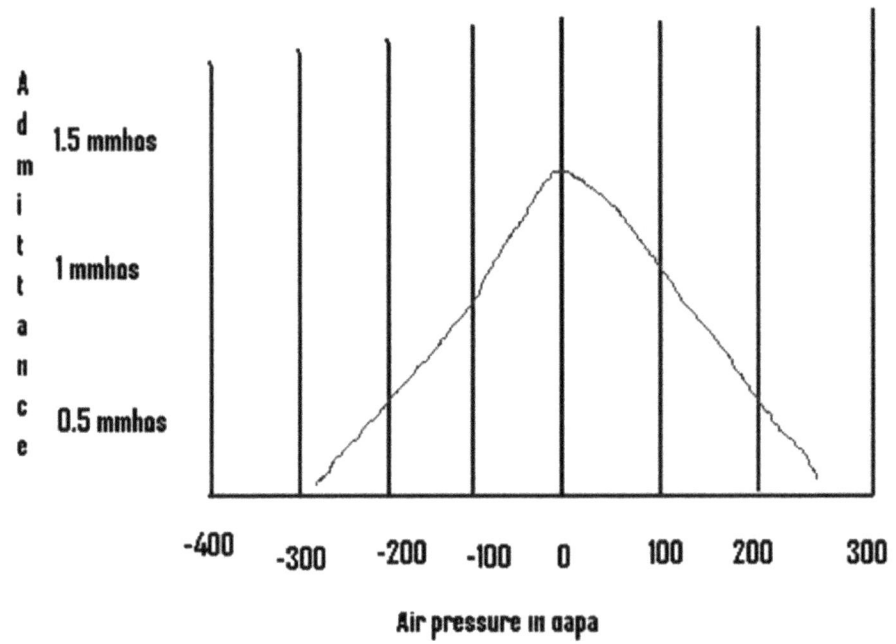

Type B tympanogram

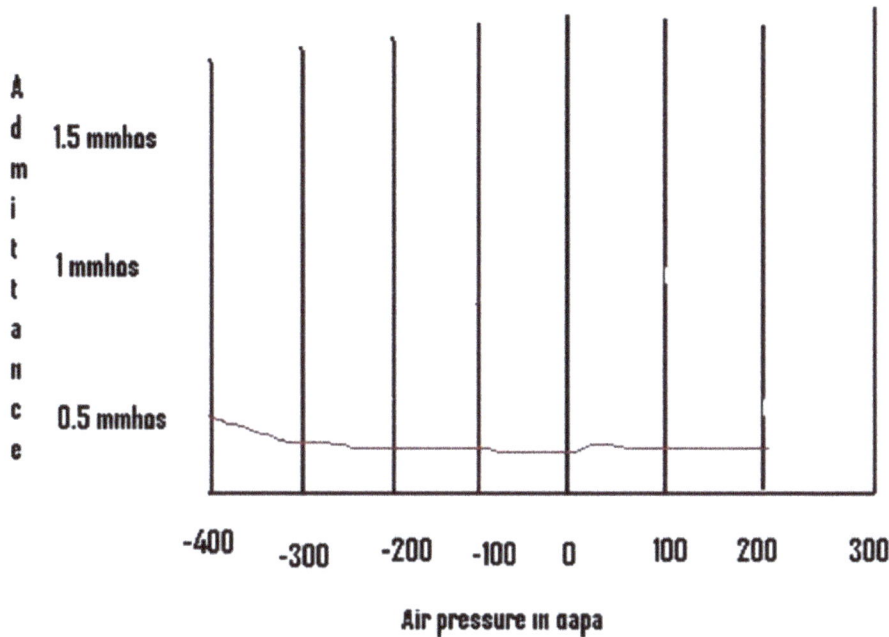

Type C tympanogram

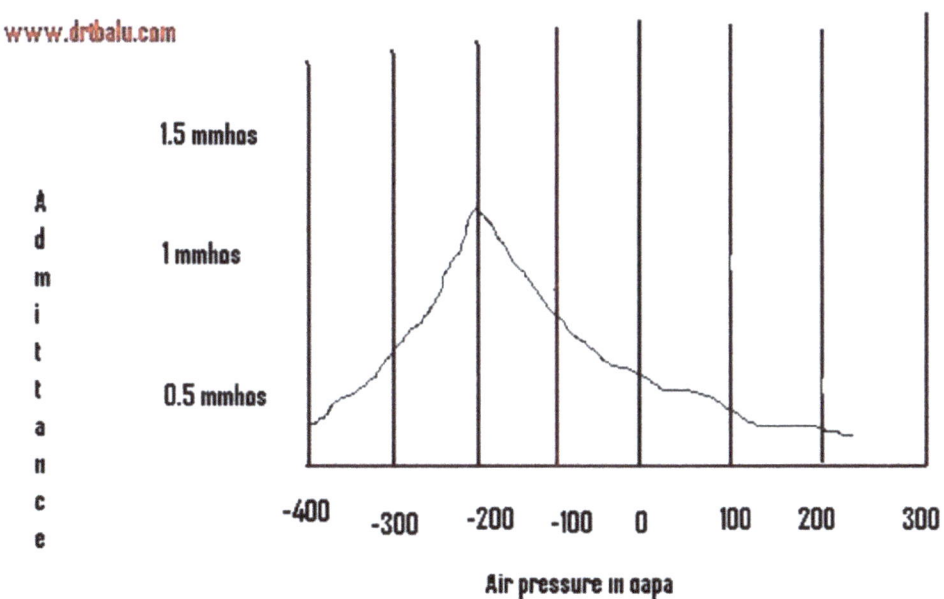

Tympanograms are categorized according to the shape of the plot. A normal tympanogram (left) is labeled Type A. There is a normal pressure in the middle ear with normal mobility of the eardrum and ossicles. Type B and C tympanograms may reveal fluid in the middle ear, perforation of the tympanic membrane, scarring of the tympanic membrane, lack of contact between the ossicles, or a tumor in the middle ear.

The categorising of tympanometric data should not be used as a diagnostic indicator. It is merely a description of shape. There is no clear distinction between the three types, nor the two subtypes of type A, namely A S and A D. Only measures of static acoustic admittance, ear canal volume, and tympanometric width/gradient compared to sex, age, and race specific normative data can be used to somewhat accurately diagnose middle ear pathology along with the use of other audiometric data (e.g. air and bone conduction thresholds, otoscopic examination, normal word recognition at elevated presentation levels, etc.).

An otoacoustic emission (OAE) is a sound which is generated from within the inner ear.

Having been predicted by Thomas Gold in 1948, its existence was first demonstrated experimentally by David Kemp in 1978—and otoacoustic emissions have since been shown to arise through a number of different cellular and mechanical causes within the inner ear. Studies have shown that OAEs disappear after the inner ear has been damaged, so OAEs are often used in the laboratory and the clinic as a measure of inner ear health. There are two types of otoacoustic emissions: spontaneous otoacoustic emissions (SOAEs), which can occur without external stimulation, and evoked otoacoustic emissions (EOAEs), which require an evoking stimulus. OAEs are considered to be related to the amplification function of the cochlea. In the absence of external stimulation, the activity of the cochlear amplifier increases, leading to the production of sound. The most common test to measure the OAEs is the Distortion Product (DPOAE) and transient evoked otoacoustic emissions (TEOAE). It has been found that distortion product otoacoustic emissions (DPOAEs) have provided the most information for detecting mild hearing loss in high frequencies when compared to transient evoked otoacoustic emissions (TEOAE). DPOAEs can help with detecting an early onset of noise-induced hearing loss.

Otoacoustic Emissions
Objective measure of the integrity and function of the outer-hair cells of the cochlea. Results report the present or absent of thresholds per frequencies and per ear in a normal hearing patient.

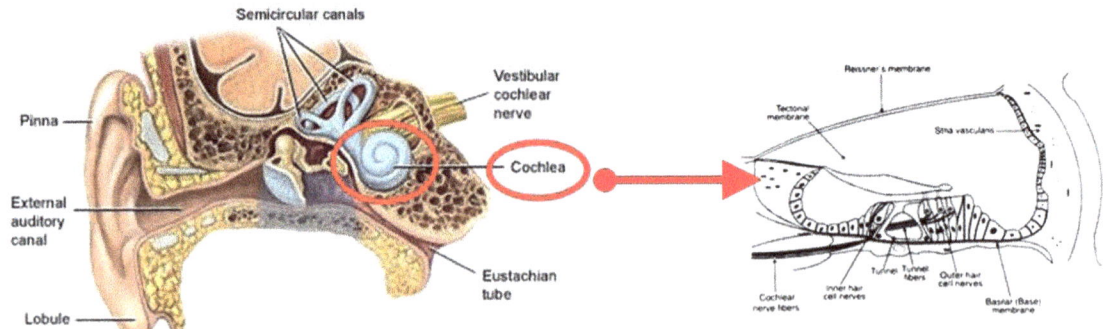

What Does the DPOAE Measurement Look Like?

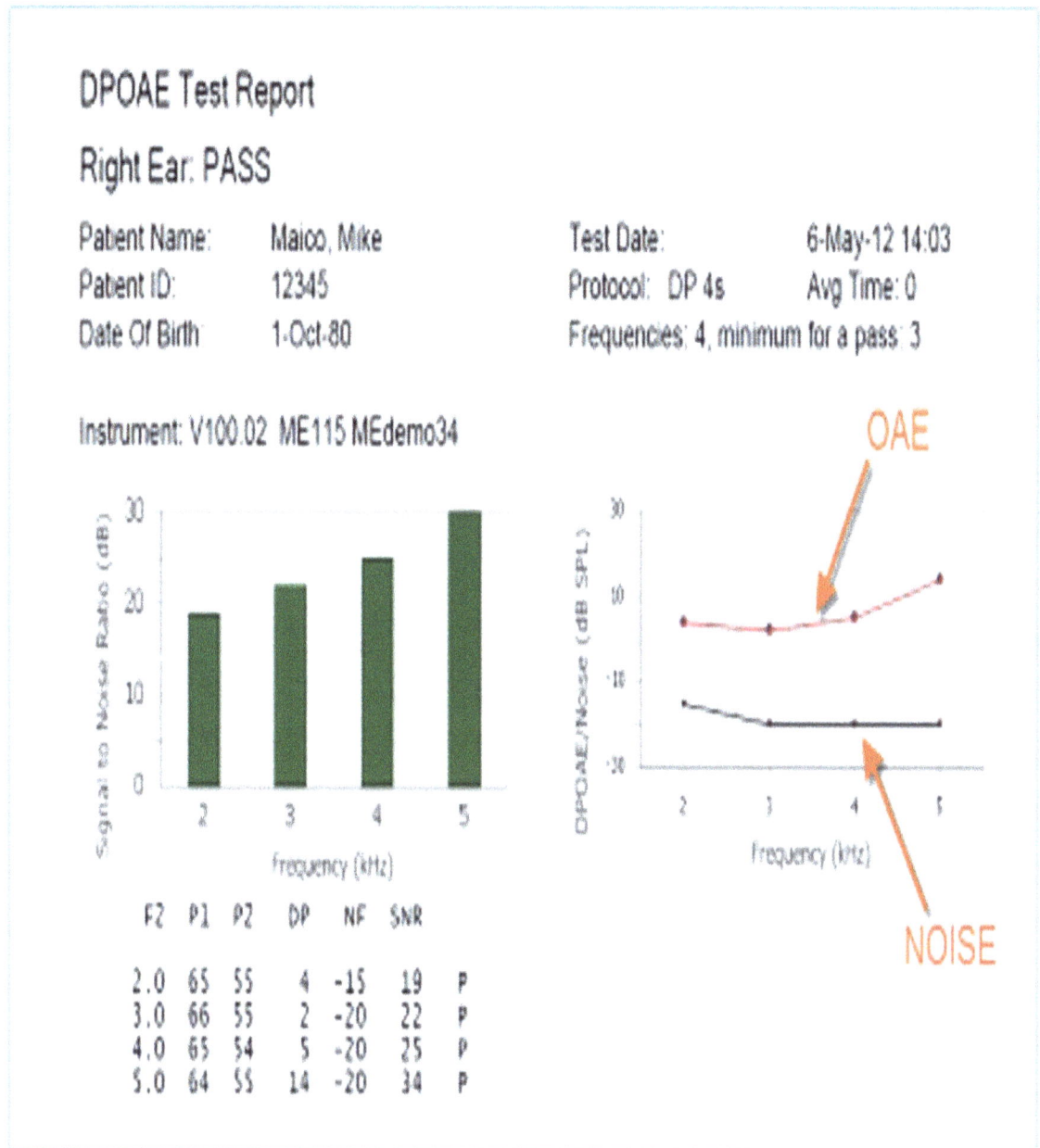

VNG

Videonystagmography (VNG) technologies for testing inner ear and central motor functions. VNG testing is considered the new standard for testing inner ear functions over Electronystagmography (ENG), because VNG measures the movements of the eyes directly through infrared cameras, instead of measuring the mastoid muscles around the eyes with electrodes like the previous ENG version. VNG testing is more accurate, more consistent, and more comfortable for the patient. By having the patient more comfortable and relaxed, consistent and accurate test results are more easily achieved.

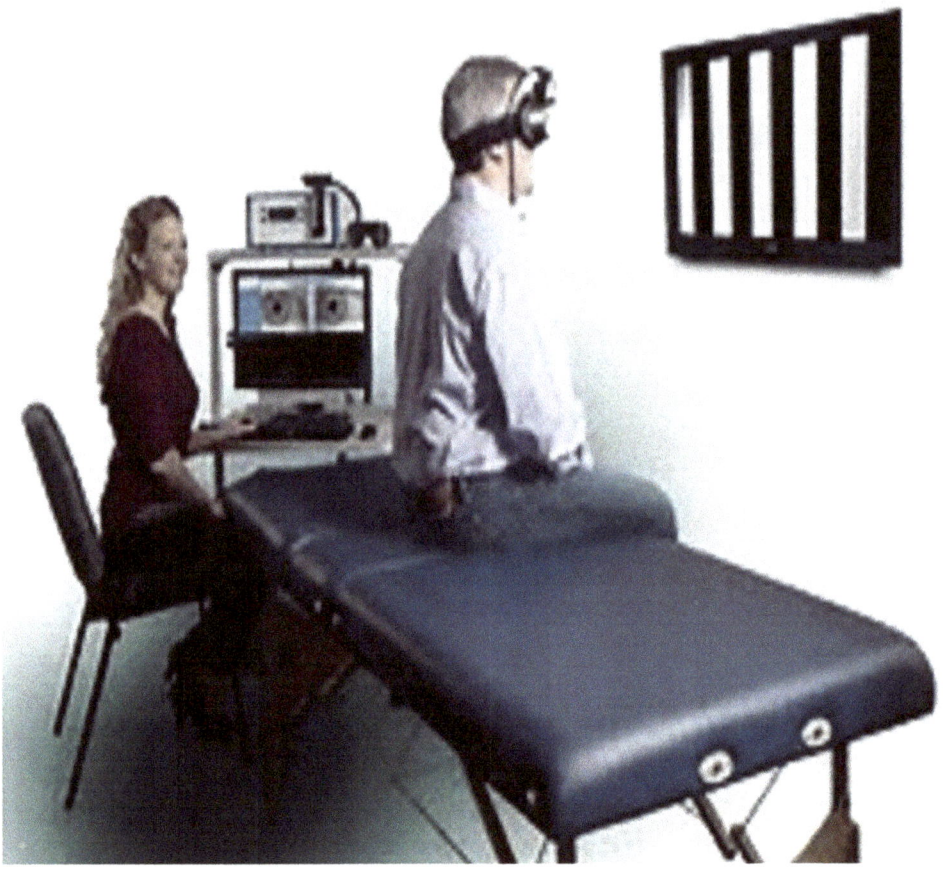

VNG testing is used to determine if a vestibular (inner ear) disease may be causing a balance or dizziness problem, and is one of the only tests available today that can decipher between a unilateral (one ear) and bilateral (both ears) vestibular loss. VNG testing is a battery of tests designed to document the patient's ability to follow visual objects with their eyes and how well the eyes respond to information from the vestibular system.

VNG Report
Testing Protocols: Spontaneous gaze, up/down/left/right directional gaze, gaze with fixation, 30 degrees. Saccades test, horizontal and vertical head rotation tests, torsion swing with or without fixation tests, high-frequency head shake, positional tests, bi-directional Optokinetic test, left/right Dix-Hallpike maneuver and bithermal calorics

Results:
Spontaneous Gaze: Describe random eye movements.

Gaze w/Fixation: Describe if suppression is Normal during fixation.

Saccades: Latency: Describes if the eye movement velocities and accuracies are normal.

Optokinetic: Describe normal optokinetic nystagmus is identified in both the horizontal and vertical plane.

Directional Gaze: describes that no clear nystagmus processes are identified in the up, down, left, or right gaze directions.

Horizontal/Vertical Head Rotation: Describes normal evoked nystagmus.

Suppression test: Normal suppression of evoked nystagmus with fixation.

High-Frequency Head Shake: Describes if nystagmus is present in both Right and left direction and up beating and down beating.

Dix-Hallpike: describes if their nystagmus present in head hanging in either right or left to diagnosis of BPPV.

Positional Tests: describes if nystagmus is present in various test positions.

Bithermal Calorics: Caloric irrigations of both warm and cold to determine if there is a weakness in the either ear. This reported by percent of weakness.

Vertigo

Endolymphatic Hydrops (Ménière Syndrome)

Increase endolymphatic fluid on the compartment of the inner ear causing excessive pressure on the labyrinth causing vertiginous bouts that can last hours, low frequency sensorineural hearing loss or fluctuating hearing, sensation of aural fullness and Tinnitus (low tone and blowing). Most commonly unilaterally, however, it can be bilateral. Audiogram with demonstrate a low frequency sensoneural hearing loss and ENG/VNG Caloric test will demonstrate a loss or impairment of thermally induced nystagmus on the affected side. The two most common causes are head trauma and syphilis. Primary treatment involves vestibular suppressant medication, diuretic (Acetazolamide), and low-salt diet. For refractory cases, patient will undergo intratympanic corticosteroids injections, endolymphatic sac decompression, vestibular ablation via transtympanic gentamycin injections, vestibular nerve resection, or surgical labyrinthectomy.

Labyrinthitis

Causes can be viral, syphilis, mycotic, keratoma, peripheral fistulas, Herpes Zoster, and bacteria. Bacterial infection needs to be treated with antibiotic if fever is involved. The onset is an acute severe dissibilitating vertigo lasting several days to a week with accompanied by hearing loss and tinnitus and if bacterial fever. The hearing loss and tinnitus may recover over the next six weeks in the involved ear. With mumps, the loss can be permanent. The hearing loss on the Audiogram can involve all the frequencies, however, most common is low frequencies. ENG/VNG Caloric test will demonstrate a loss or impairment of thermally induced nystagmus on the affected side. Treatment consist of vestibular suppressants, antibiotics if bacterial; if mycotic, antifungal; if Herpes Zoster, antiviral and high dose prednisone with all for one week.

Vestibular Neuronitis
This is a paroxysmal usually single bout of vertigo which is without accompanying impairment of the auditory function. The bout usually lasts several days to a week and is not as violent as a labyrinthitis bout. The cause of this disorder is unknown however it is presumed to be a post viral infection. Audiogram would be normal or have no change from prior audiogram. ENG/VNG caloric test will demonstrate an absent response to the caloric stimulation of the affected ear or both if both ears are affected. A treatment consists of vestibular suppressants and high dose prednisone for a week.

Benign Paroxysmal Positioning Vertigo (BPPV)
This type of vertigo is a recurrent vertiginous bout lasting less than a minute which is provoked by changes in head position rather than changes in posture. The cause of BPPV occur with otoconia from the utricle fragment and converge into the horizontal and vertical canals causing excitatory stimulation sending erroneous information to the vestibular nucleus causing the catch-up nystagmus to occur. This is usually seen on the Dix-Hallpike maneuver. The Auditory function and ENG/VNG Caloric is not affected. Some central lesions can mimic positioning vertigo via vertebrobasillar insufficiency and an MRI is warranted to r/o central lesions. In Central lesions there is latent period, fatigability or habituation of symptoms. Treatment of BPPV involves Vestibular Rehabilitation (Epley maneuver or the Brandt-Daroff exercise) so as move the otoconia from the semicircular canals. No vestibular suppressant is effective and should not be used.

Perilymphatic Fistula
This occurs when a leakage of the perilymphatic fluid from the inner ear leakages into the tympanic cavity via tear or rupture of the round or oval window producing vertigo and sudden hearing loss. The causes are from head trauma, extreme barotraumas from air flights or scuba diving, vigorous Valsalva maneuver and Weight lifting. The vertiginous bouts can last seconds to minutes. The Audiogram will demonstrate a significant to profound SNHL of the affected ear. ENG/VNG caloric test will demonstrate an absent response to the caloric stimulation of the affected ear or both if both ears are affected. Treatment is exploratory surgery of the middle ear with graph tissue repair.

Superior Semicircular Canal Dehiscence (SSCD)
This occurs when there is a small congenital deficiency in the bony covering of the lateral portion of the superior semicircular canal. Vertigo is elicited by loud sound, straining and pressure on the labyrinth during a conductive hearing impairment. The vertiginous boat can last days. Audiogram will demonstrate a minor conductive hearing loss with normal tympagrams. ENG/VNG caloric testing would not demonstrate any weakness or directional preponderance. The VEMP would positive in the affected

ear. High resolution mm coronal cuts CT would demonstrate the absence of bone at the site of the dehiscence. The treatment would be a lateral surgical approach and sealing the dehiscent canal.

Cervical Vertigo

This occurs when the neck is hyperextended as the eye focuses upward and is elicited after a neck injury or degenerative cervical spine disease. Positional receptors located in the facets of the cervical spine are important physiologically in the coordination of head and eye movement. The vertiginous bout is brief, lasting seconds to a minute. The Audiogram would be normal as well as the ENG/VNG calories. Treatment is neck exercise and manipulation of the spine.

Migraines Vertigo

This is one of the multiple symptoms of Migraine. The vertiginous bout can last days (as long as the migraine lasts). The vertigo does not affect the Auditory or vestibular function. Management is accomplished by treating the Migraine Headache.

Central Lesion Vertigo

The Cerebellopontine angle (CP) is bounded by the pons, the cerebellum, and the Temporal bone. The seventh (7th) and eight (8th) CN nerves leave the pons, runs through the angle, and enter the temporal bone by way of the internal auditory canal (IAC). The tumor of the Cerebellopontine angle usually produces a slow, progressive loss of vestibular function and of the hearing without episodic vertigo. The fifth (5th) and seventh (7th) CN are commonly involved, causing ipsilateral facial numbness and weakness. In the later stages of progression, involvement of the sixth (6th) and ninth (9th) and tenth (10th) CN given rise to Diplopia, Dysphonia, and Dysphagia. As the tumors grows, it causes compression of the brain stem and cerebellum resulting in ipsilateral gaze dysfunction and dysmetria of the extremities. Audiograms reveal a SNHL, impaired Speech Discrimination, tone decay, and loss of stapedius reflex on the affected side. ENG/VNG calories reveal loss of vestibular function on the affected side. CT usually reveals erosion of the medial lip of the IAC. Treatment is Surgical or Cyber Knife

ABR Testing

The procedure for ABR is very simple. The patient relaxes in a darkened room. The duration of the test is 20-60 minutes. The time varies depending on patient and what information the physician is seeking. There are typically four surface/skin electrodes used. Two are placed on the center of the forehead, one above the other about 2 inches apart. The top electrode may be placed on the top of the head (but this can get messy). The remaining electrodes are placed one on each ear lobe or behind the ear on the boney bump (mastoid bone). Insert earphones are placed in each ear, and the patient is instructed to close the eyes and relax during the test. Typically, the lights in the room are turned off to minimize external electrical interference. The patient hears a clicking sound during testing. Sometimes in the opposite ear there will be a static, or white noise. Depending on the bio-electric noise, or internal body noise, the collection of information may go quickly or take a little time. A graphic pattern is produce as shown below.

ABR Electrode Montage

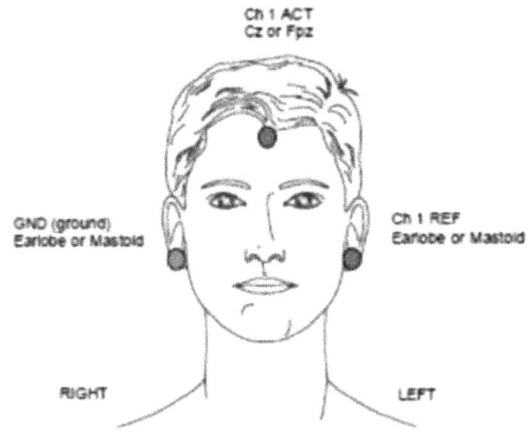

AUDITORY BRAINSTEM RESPONSE MONTAGES

1-Channel ABR
ELECTRODE SWITCHING ON

ABR Tracing Patterns

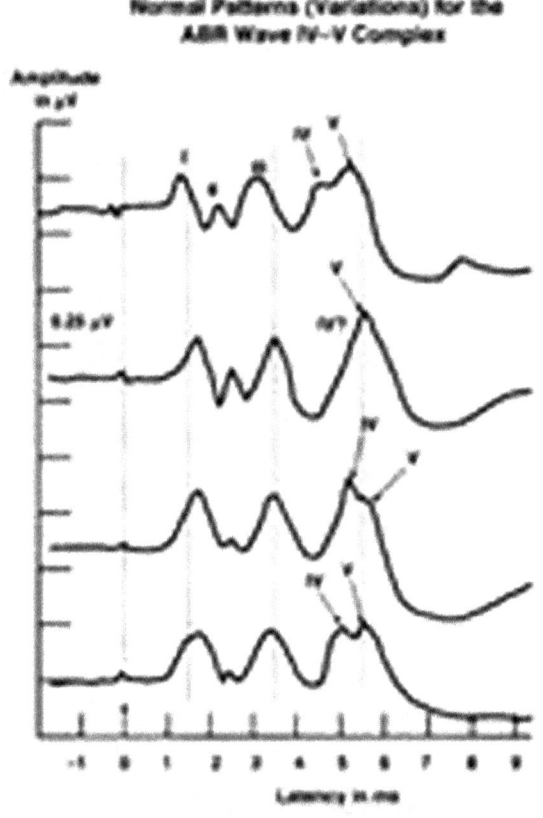

Normal Patterns (Variations) for the
ABR Wave IV~V Complex

The basic ABR wave form is shown in the picture above. Each of the numbered peaks represents specific locations along cranial nerve VIII, or acoustic nerve, and lower brainstem. These peaks should appear in a specific time pattern. Waves I and II provide information regarding the auditory nerve as it is leaving the cochlea and can help in diagnosing auditory neuropathy/dys-synchrony (Central Auditory Processing Disorder). Waves III through V provide information about the transmission of neural impulses through the lower brainstem. Wave V is considered the most clinically useful wave. The timing of this wave can be of significant importance when trying to determine retro-cochlear pathology, such as acoustic neuroma or vestibular schwannoma, a benign growth on the cranial nerve eight.

Neurological ABR Report Sample

Brainstem Auditory Evoked Potential Study: Independent stimulation of the left and right ears with rarefaction clicks and other stimulating and recording parameters standardized for this laboratory showed definite reproducible waveforms. On left-sided stimulation, at 100 dB interpeak latencies were as follows: I-III 2.2 msec, III-V 2.04 msec, I-V 4.24 msec. On right-sided stimulation, this was measured as follows: I-III 2.2 msec, III-V 2.06 msec, I-V 4.26 msec. These are within normal limits. The neurological ABR is measuring delay between both ears to determine if there is a retrocochlear lesion to the eighth nerve. (Ie Acoustic Neuroma/schwannoma)

Neurological ABR Tracing sample

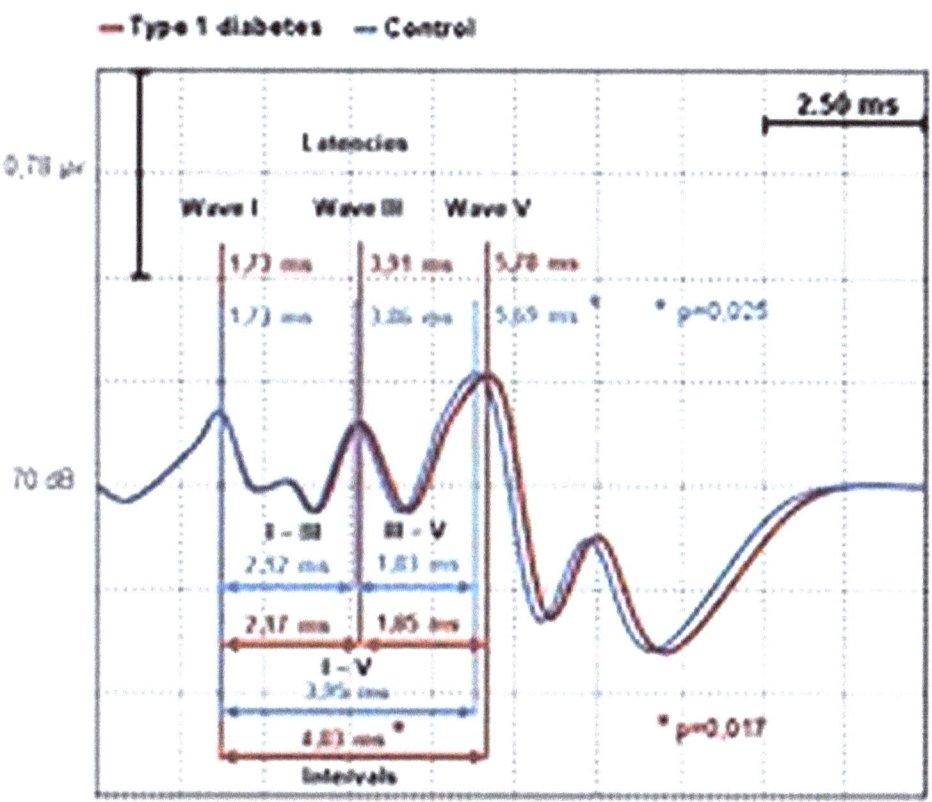

Location of ABR Wave from Cochlea to Auditory Cortex

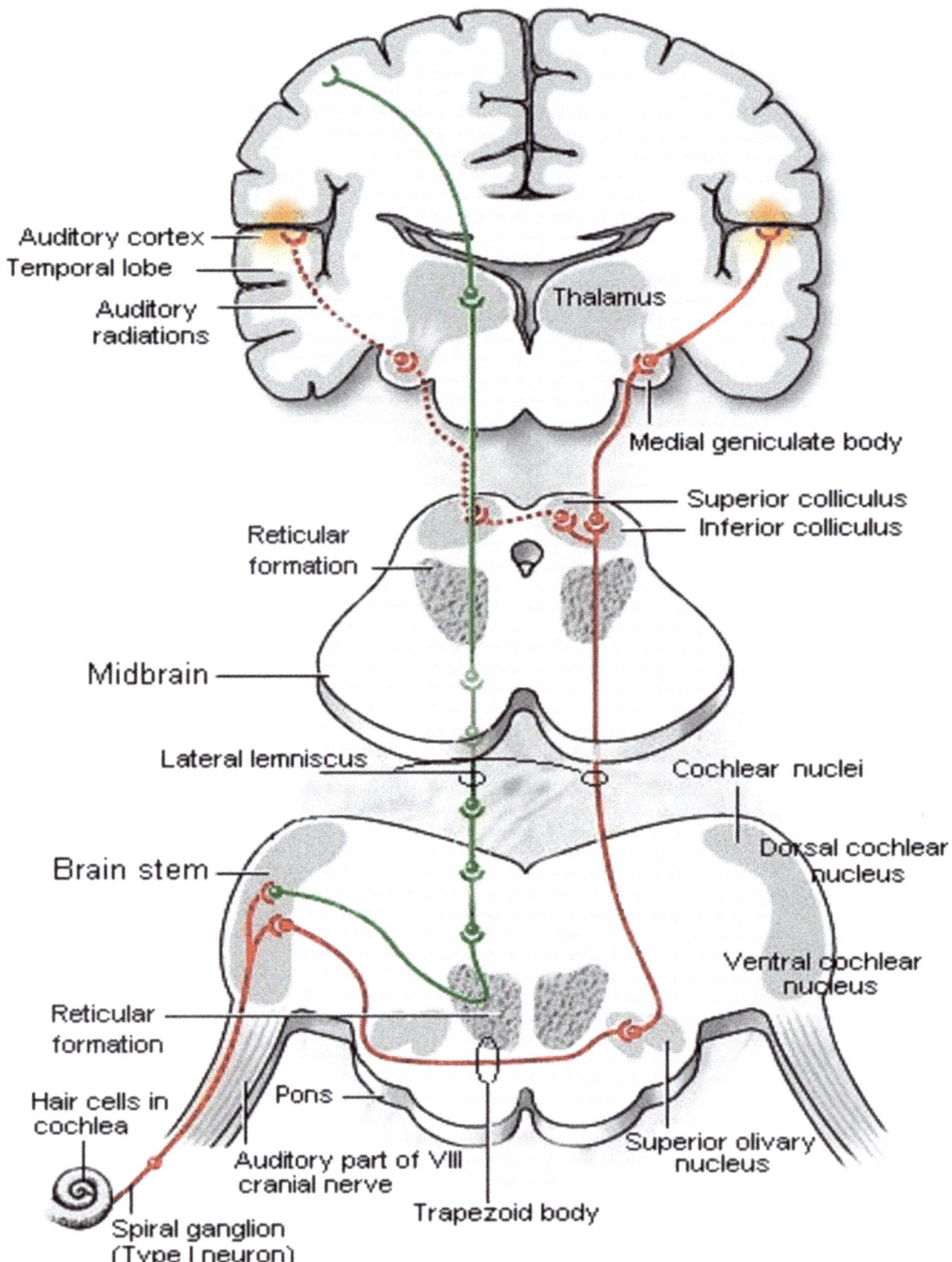

Side of Lesion

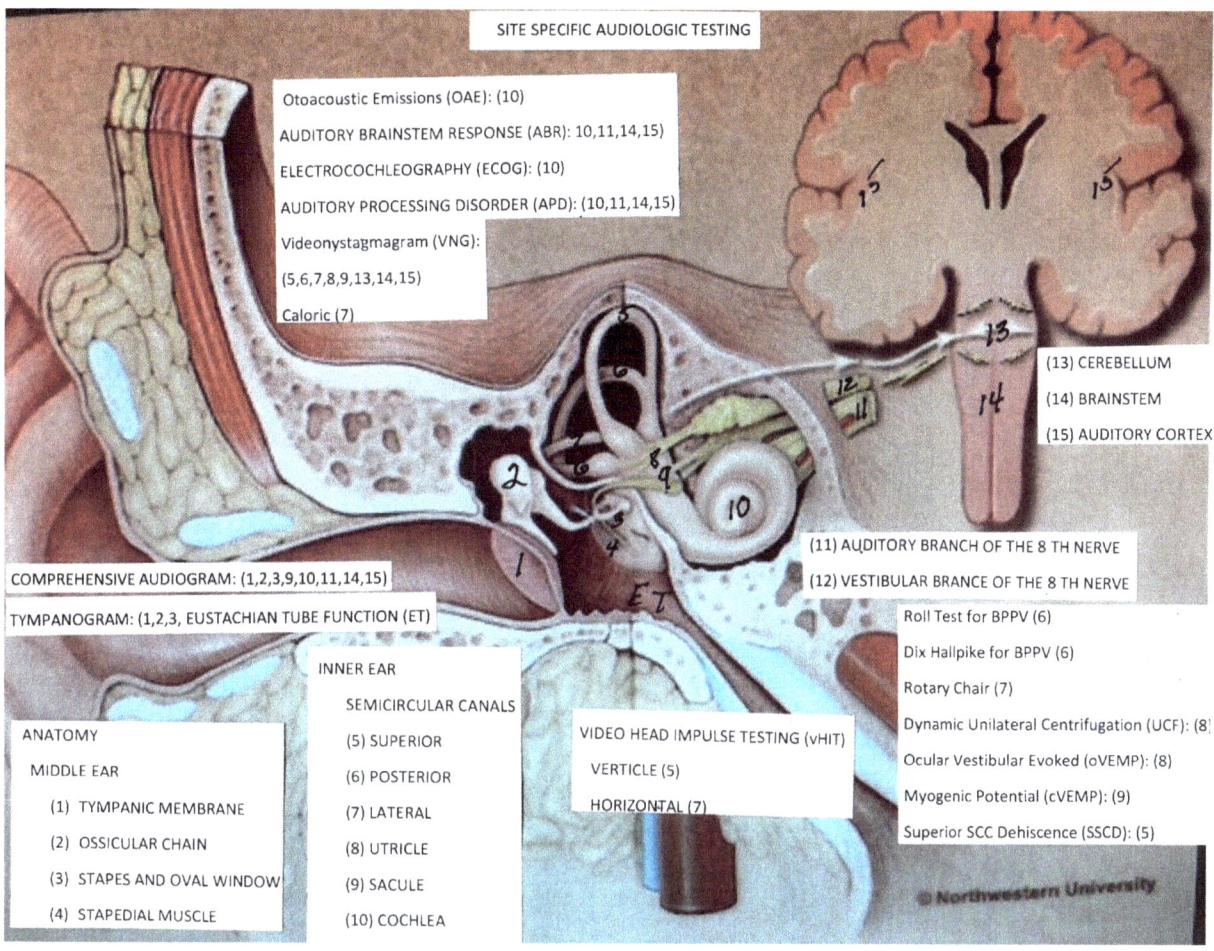

SITE SPECIFIC AUDIOLOGIC TESTING

Otoacoustic Emissions (OAE): (10)

AUDITORY BRAINSTEM RESPONSE (ABR): 10,11,14,15)

ELECTROCOCHLEOGRAPHY (ECOG): (10)

AUDITORY PROCESSING DISORDER (APD): (10,11,14,15)

Videonystagmagram (VNG):
(5,6,7,8,9,13,14,15)

Caloric (7)

(13) CEREBELLUM

(14) BRAINSTEM

(15) AUDITORY CORTEX

(11) AUDITORY BRANCH OF THE 8 TH NERVE

(12) VESTIBULAR BRANCE OF THE 8 TH NERVE

COMPREHENSIVE AUDIOGRAM: (1,2,3,9,10,11,14,15)

TYMPANOGRAM: (1,2,3, EUSTACHIAN TUBE FUNCTION (ET)

ANATOMY

MIDDLE EAR

(1) TYMPANIC MEMBRANE

(2) OSSICULAR CHAIN

(3) STAPES AND OVAL WINDOW

(4) STAPEDIAL MUSCLE

INNER EAR

SEMICIRCULAR CANALS

(5) SUPERIOR

(6) POSTERIOR

(7) LATERAL

(8) UTRICLE

(9) SACULE

(10) COCHLEA

VIDEO HEAD IMPULSE TESTING (vHIT)

VERTICLE (5)

HORIZONTAL (7)

Roll Test for BPPV (6)

Dix Hallpike for BPPV (6)

Rotary Chair (7)

Dynamic Unilateral Centrifugation (UCF): (8)

Ocular Vestibular Evoked (oVEMP): (8)

Myogenic Potential (cVEMP): (9)

Superior SCC Dehiscence (SSCD): (5)

© Northwestern University

Chapter Three
Abnormal Findings

Most common symptoms reported from patient are Tinnitus, vertigo and dizziness, otalgia, persistent ear fullness (after a flight/diving), abnormal sensitivity to sound (sound seems too loud), wax impaction, decrease hearing, infection of ears, bleeding from the ear, chronic drainage from ear canal, trauma to the ear with hearing loss and/or dizziness, hearing their voice, loss of hearing acuity after taking medication or chemotherapy, baby failed new born screening and sudden hearing loss. As a clinical provider, your task to learn and understand the types of audiometric testing need to provide the patient with a reason and possible cure for their hearing disorder. Let's review causes of hearing loss and their audiometric data.

Types of Hearing loss
- Hearing Loss is described as a range
- Ranges from Mild through Profound

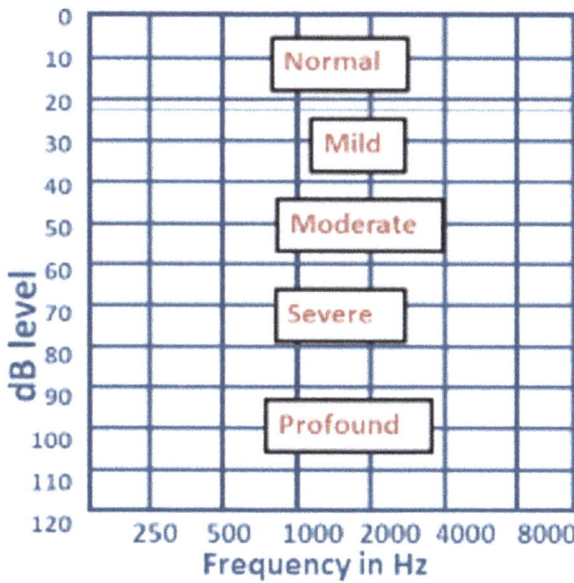

The following section is based on abnormal conditions of the external, middle, inner ear and brainstem and auditory cortex.

We will begin with the pinna to the auditory cortex and what test to request to verify the site of lesion that is causing the hearing disorder.

The Pinna

The pinna contributes about 10 dB to the auditory system so any deformity (Microtia) or absence (Anotia) of the pinna would cause hearing loss. Audiogram with this type of loss would demonstrate a conductive loss, and the patient would be tested via Bone Conduction.

External Auditory Canal (EAC)

Disorder of the EAC can be caused by congenital atresia were portions of the cartilaginous portion of the EAC fails to develop partially or not at all, stenosis of the EAC, Foreign body, Cerumen impaction, exotomas, otitis externa, and congenital abnormalities. The amplification of sound by the EAC has an increase in level of about 15 to 25 dB in a frequency range of 1.5 kHz to 7 kHz. Children with Treacher Collins Syndrome usually have bilateral Atresia, however normally it presents in one of the ears. Audiogram will demonstrate a mild conduction hearing loss.

The Tympanic Membrane (TM)

Disorders of the TM can be caused from obstruction of the mobility of the TM from wax impactions, infection, sclerosis of the TM membrane, TM perforation, middle ear pathology, and congenital abnormalities. The TM can be evaluated by both an audiogram and tympanogram. The audiogram will demonstrate a mild conductive hearing loss with airborne gaps. The Tympanogram will have an array of results depending on the TM status. (See Tympanometry tracings). A type A indicates normal TM, Type As is a stiff TM which can be sclerosis, early otosclerosis of stapes, cerumen and tumor of the EAC. A type AS can be caused by a flaccid TM or disarticulation of the Ossicular Chain from trauma. Type C is indicative of excessive negative or positive pressure in the middle ear which is caused by the process of infection or Eustachian Tube Dysfunction (ETD). Type B is complete stiffness of the TM cause by infected and sterile middle ear effusion from ETD or Mastoiditis.

Type A

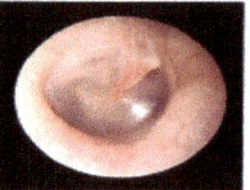

- Normal middle ear pressure
- Normal eardrum movement
- Normal ear canal volume

Example:

➤ Normal middle ear

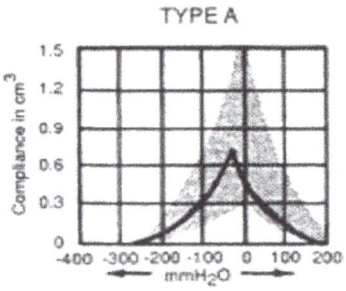

Type A$_s$

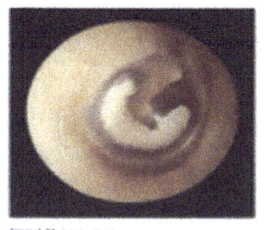

- Reduced Compliance
- Normal Middle-ear pressure
- Normal ear canal volume

Example:

➢ Fixation of ossicles

➢ Scarring on TM

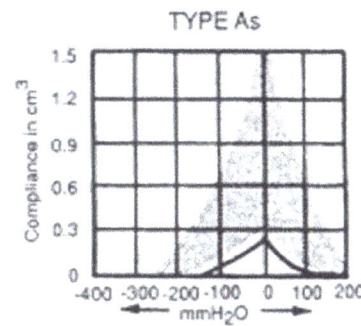

Type B (normal volume)

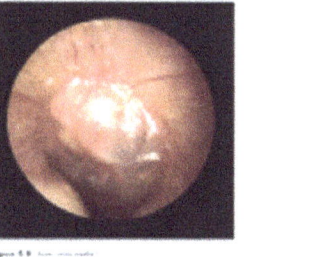

- "Flat"
- No compliance or pressure peak indicated
- <u>Normal</u> ear canal volume

Example:

➢ Middle-ear fluid

Type B (increased volume)

- "Flat"
- No compliance or pressure peak indicated
- Increased ear canal volume

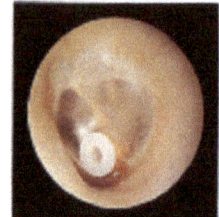 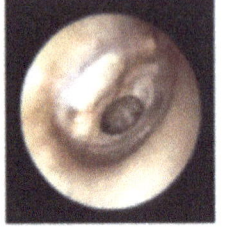

TYPE B

Example:

➢ Perforated TM
➢ Patent P.E. Tubes

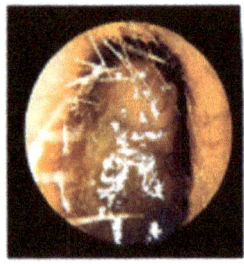

Type B (decreased volume)

- "Flat"
- No compliance or pressure peak indicated
- Decreased ear canal volume

TYPE B

Example:

➢ Occluding Wax
➢ Probe up against canal wall??

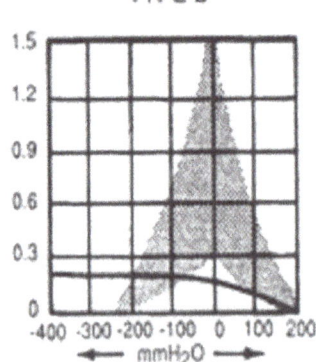

Middle Ear (ME)

Disorder of the ME causes conductive hearing loss due to abnormalities of the structure or function of the middle ear in direct relationship to the amount of the disease in the ME. The ME can attribute 25 to 30 dB of increased hearing. Causes of ME disorder is Otitis Media, Eustachian Tube Dysfunction, Patulous Eustachian Tube, Tympanosclerosis, Chronic Mastoid disease, Ossicular Chain Dysfunction/disarticulation, Cholesteatoma, surgical changes of the TM (Myringotomy and tympanoplasty), OC (stapedectomy), Mastoidectomy, and congenital abnormalities.

Audiological Testing of the ME in Audiogram, OAE, Tympanograms, ABR and CAT SCAN. (See Audiogram, OAE results if the conductive process is mild), ABR tracing demonstrating latency disorder. CT is used to corroborate the audiometric data.

Inner Ear

The inner ear is a fluid filled membranous organ call the labyrinth and divided into the cochlea, which interfaces between the middle ear, and the auditory nerve. The inner ear converts sounds into a form of electro-chemical energy that transmits information in terms of their frequency, intensity and phase to the brainstem to the auditory cortex. The vestibular portion of the inner ear transmits information to the brain data pertaining to patient's position and movement. Any lesion in either organ will produce a sensorineuro hearing loss since it's composed of sensory and nerve cells. A conductive component of the audiometric testing would demonstrate a fistula in the fluid filled membranous organ. The audiogram will demonstrate a conductive hearing loss with normal Tympanograms, abnormal VEMP, ECOG, and VNG results. However, this is rare, and 99% of the time is Sensorineural Hearing loss. Causes of abnormal inner ear sensorineural hearing loss occur at the Cochlea portion of the inner ear the results are a combination of sensorineural hearing loss and dysacusis (inability to understand speech) and bone conduction and air conduction results interweave on the audiogram and speech discrimination generally becomes poorer in direct relationship to the amount of hearing loss. Common causes of injury to the inner ear are ototoxic drugs, noise-induced hearing loss, viral and bacterial diseases (Cytomegalovirus [CMV], Syphilis, Rubella, Toxoplasmosis, Herpes simplex virus, Mumps, Measles, Bacterial Meningitis, and Herpes Zoster Oticus), Genetic Disorder and end stage Ménière's Disease.

Ototoxic drugs cause inner ear hearing loss (SNHL). The amount of damage to the inner ear is dependent on the duration and dosage used. Some ototoxic-induced hearing losses are reversible to stoppage of use i.e. Loop Diuretics, Salicylates and Quinine. Ototoxic Drugs such as Aminoglycosides, Antibiotics, and Chemotherapy are not reversible and, during their use, are closely monitor audiometrically. Since Ototoxicity initially effects the high frequencies most, audiologists conduct high frequency audiometry from 10 kHz 18 kHz to closely monitor early changes in the patient's hearing.

Central Hearing Impairment

Tumors, degenerative nerve diseases, and genetic syndromes are responsible for central hearing impairments. Central hearing impairment is cause by lesions in the cortex. There are two types of central hearing loss in infants and children. Auditory Processing Disorder (APD) which is a disorder that affects the way the brain processes auditory information via an acquired auditory processing disorder, hereditary, and genetic characteristics of central auditory processing disorder. Infants and children with APD usually have normal structure and function of the outer, middle, and inner ear of the peripheral hearing system; however, they cannot process the information they hear in the same way as other normal-hearing children. This leads to difficulties in recognizing and interpreting sounds of normal speech. You will have a normal audiogram with very poor speech test results.

Auditory Neuropathy (AN) is a variety of hearing loss in which the outer hair cells within the cochlea are present and functional, but sound information is not transmitted to the auditory nerve and brain properly. Infants at risk for developing auditory neuropathy include infants with hypoxia, prematurity, neurologic impairment, hyperbilirubinemia, or neonates who spend a long period in the neonatal intensive care unit (NICU). You will have a normal OAE and Abnormal ABR. In adults, the impairments are neurologic disorders such as Multiple Sclerosis and benign and malignant tumors of the brain, and vascular accidents.

Hereditary Hearing Loss

Hearing disorders cause by hereditary hearing loss are classified in two groups, exogenous and endogenous. Exogenous hearing disorders are those cause by toxicity, noise, head trauma, and injury to the inner ear.

Endogenous hearing disorders are hereditary. The endogenous hearing disorder is transmitted to the fetus as an inherited gene trait. There are three modes of transmission for hereditary hearing loss. Autosomal recessive (implies that the abnormal gene is not carried on the sex chromosomes), autorecessive inheritance (one parent carries the abnormal gene and the trait has a 50% chance of being transmitted to the child), and X-linked (gene is determined by genes located on the sex linked X chromosomes). The X-linked occurs in about 2-3% of hereditary hearing loss. It is estimated that there are over 400 different genes syndrome which cause various types of hearing disorders. However, 70% of hereditary hearing loss is nonsyndromic. Type of autosomal syndrome associated with hearing loss is Waardenburg Syndrome, branchio-otorenal syndrome and neurofibromatosis 2 (NF2). Autorecessive syndromes are Usher syndrome and Pendred syndrome. X-linked inheritance is Alport syndrome. The type of hearing loss varies with the syndrome (see attached most common syndrome associated with hearing loss). To learn more on genetics and hearing loss, go to http://www.ncbi.nlm.nih.gov.

Syndromes with hearing loss

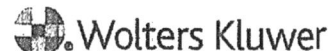

Selected syndromes associated with hearing loss

Syndrome	Features	Caused by mutation	Sensorineural	Conductive	Mixed
Waardenburg syndrome (AD)	White forelock, heterochromic irides, broad mandible, deafness	X	X		
Usher syndrome (AR)	Retinitis pigmentosa, ataxia, deafness	X	X		
Pendred syndrome (AR)	Familial goiter, dysfunctional iodide organization, deafness	X	X		
Alport syndrome (XL, AR, AD)	Nephritis, deafness, lens, defects, retinitis	X	X		
Craniofacial anomalies (eg, Apert syndrome, Pfeiffer syndrome, Crouzon syndrome)	Craniosynostosis, micrognathia, syndactyly		X	X	X
CHARGE (AD, isolated cases)	Choanal atresia, colobomas, heart defect, intellectual disability, genital hypoplasia, ear anomalies, deafness	X	X		X
Hemifacial microsomia (oculo-auriculo-vertebral spectrum, Goldenhar syndrome) (sporadic, AD)	Facial hypoplasia, ear anomalies, hemivertibrae, parotid gland dysfunction	X		X	X
Mucopolysaccharidosis Hurler (AR), Hunter (XL), Maroteaux-Lamy (AR)	Coarse facies, stiff joints, intellectual disability, cloudy corneas	X			X
Treacher-Collins syndrome (AD)	Facial malformation, cleft palate, deafness	X		X	

Syndromes with hearing loss

Syndrome	Features				
Otopalatodigital syndrome (XL)	Deafness, cleft palate, broad digits			X	
Stickler syndrome (AD)	Cleft palate, micrognathia, myopia, cataracts, spondyloepiphyseal dysplasia, deafness	X		X	
LEOPARD syndrome (AD)	Multiple lentigenes, pulmonic stenosis, hypertelorism, deafness, genital anomalies	X	X		
Kartagener syndrome (AR)	Situs inversus, immobile cilia, heart defects, splenic anomalies, deafness	X			
Cockayne syndrome (AR)	Retinal degeneration, senile-like changes, growth retardation, photosensitivity, deafness	X	X		
Achondroplasia (AD)	Short limbs, hydrocephalus	X			X
Branchiootorenal syndrome (AD)	Branchial anomalies, ear malformations, renal anomalies	X	X	X	X
Klippel-Feil syndrome (sporadic, AD, AR)	Fused cervical vertebrae, webbed neck, deafness, congenital heart defect		X	X	X
Duane syndrome (sporadic, AD)	Ocular strabismus, ear anomalies, skeletal anomalies, cranial nerve palsies, deafness	X		X	
Marfan syndrome (AD)	Lens subluxation, arachnodactyly, aortic aneurysm, hyperextensibility, deafness	X	X	X	X
Mobius syndrome (sporadic, AD, AR)	Cranial nerve palsies, limb anomalies, hypoglossia,			X	

Syndromes with hearing loss

	micrognathia, deafness				
Muckle-Wells syndrome (AD)	Amyloid nephropathy, urticaria, deafness	X	X		
Pierre-Robin syndrome (AR, XL)	Micrognathia, cleft palate, glossoptosis, deafness			X	
Jervell and Lange-Nielsen syndrome (AR)	Long QT, deafness	X	X		
Neurofibromatosis type I (AD)	Neurofibromas, cafe-au-lait spots, optic glioma	X			
Osteogenesis imperfecta (AD, AR)	Fragile bones, blue sclera	X			X
Ehlers-Danlos (AD, AR)	Joint hyperextensibility, fragile skin	X			X

AD: autosomal dominant inheritance; AR: autosomal recessive inheritance; XL: X-linked inheritance; CHARGE: Coloboma, Heart defect, Atresia choanae (also known as choanal atresia), Retarded growth and development, Genital abnormalities, and Ear abnormalities; LEOPARD: Lentigines, Electrocardiographic conduction abnormalities, Ocular hypertelorism, Pulmonary stenosis, Abnormal genitalia, Retarded growth, Deafness.

Graphic 66758 Version 2.0

Causes of Inner Ear Disease

A vestibular schwannoma is a benign primary intracranial tumor of the myelin-forming cells of the vestibulocochlear nerve (eighth cranial nerve). A type of schwannoma, this tumor arises from the Schwann cells responsible for the myelin sheath that helps keep peripheral nerves insulated. Although it is commonly called an acoustic neuroma, this a misnomer for two reasons. First, the tumor usually arises from the vestibular division of the vestibulocochlear nerve, rather than the cochlear division. Second, it is derived from the Schwann cells of the associated nerve, rather than the actual neurons (neuromas).

Approximately 2,000 to 3,000 cases are diagnosed each year. Most recent publications suggest that the incidence of acoustic neuromas is rising because of advances in MRI scanning. A rare tumor that mimics an Acoustic Neuroma is a metastatic breast adenoma.

Sensorineural hearing loss (SNHL) is a type of hearing loss, or deafness, in which the root cause lies in the inner ear or sensory organ (cochlea and associated structures) or the vestibulocochlear nerve (cranial nerve VIII) or neural part. SNHL accounts for about 90% of hearing loss reported. SNHL is generally permanent and can be mild, moderate, severe, profound, or total. Various other descriptors can be used such as high frequency, low frequency, U-shaped, notched, peaked, or flat depending on the shape of the audiogram, the measure of hearing.

Sensory hearing loss occurs as a consequence of damaged or deficient cochlear hair cell function [Note: disputed—discuss]. The hair cells may be abnormal at birth or damaged during the lifetime of an individual. There are both external causes of damage, like noise trauma and infection, and intrinsic abnormalities, like deafness genes. A common cause or exacerbating factor in sensory hearing loss is prolonged exposure to environmental noise; for example, being in a loud workplace without wearing protection, or having headphones set to high volumes for a long period. Exposure to a very loud noise such as a bomb blast can cause noise-induced hearing loss.

Neural, or "retrocochlear," hearing loss occurs because of damage to the cochlear nerve (CVIII). This damage may affect the initiation of the nerve impulse in the cochlear nerve or the transmission of the nerve impulse along the nerve into the brainstem.

Most cases of SNHL present with a gradual deterioration of hearing thresholds occurring over years to decades. In some the loss may eventually affect large portions of the frequency range. It may be accompanied by other symptoms such as ringing in the ears (tinnitus), dizziness, or lightheadedness (vertigo). SNHL can be genetically inherited or acquired as a result from external causes like noise or disease. It may be congenital (present at birth) or develop later in life. The most common kind of sensorineural hearing loss is age-related (presbycusis), followed by noise-induced hearing loss (NIHL).

Frequent symptoms of SNHL are loss of acuity in distinguishing foreground voices against noisy backgrounds, difficulty understanding on the telephone, some kinds of sounds seeming excessively loud or shrill (recruitment), difficulty understanding some parts of speech (fricatives and sibilants), loss of directionality of sound, especially high frequency sounds, perception that people mumble when speaking, and difficulty understanding speech. Similar symptoms are also associated with other kinds of hearing loss; audiometry or other diagnostic tests are necessary to distinguish sensorineural hearing loss.

Identification of sensorineural hearing loss is usually made by performing a pure tone audiometry (an audiogram) in which bone conduction thresholds are measured. Tympanometry and speech audiometry may be helpful. Testing is performed by an audiologist.

There is no proven or recommended treatment or cure for SNHL; management of hearing loss is usually by hearing strategies and hearing aids. In cases of profound or total deafness, a cochlear implant is a hearing surgically implantable devise which may restore a functional level of hearing. SNHL is at least partially preventable by avoiding environmental noise, ototoxic chemicals and drugs, and head trauma, and treating or inoculating against certain triggering diseases and conditions like meningitis.

Chapter Four
Hearing Disorders and Audiogram Interpretation

The primary purpose of this chapter is to provide you with a basic understanding of hearing disorders, characteristics of the hearing loss, and, most importantly, the audiometric configuration that is most closely associated to the disorder. The goal is not for you to memorize every possible disorder, along with the audiometric pattern, but when you are finished reading this chapter you should have a better understanding of how the results of the hearing test relate to the diagnosis of some common hearing disorders.

The first thing you need to know about hearing disorders is that it is critical to have a good understanding of when to refer a patient to a physician for a medical evaluation. In fact, before you even begin to discuss hearing aids with a patient it is imperative that you have ruled out a treatable medical problem involving the auditory system. This means that you have to recognize what a hearing disorder looks like on an audiogram. Before reviewing the various types of hearing disorders, let's discuss the difference between a symptom and an etiology.

Common Symptoms
The symptoms listed below are ones you will frequently encounter, and are used by physicians and audiologists on a regular basis.

Tinnitus
This is the perceived sensation of ear noise, often described as a ringing or buzzing in the ear. It is not a disorder, just the sensation to hear sounds generated by the auditory system. Tinnitus, however, is often associated with hearing loss and hearing disorders. For example, most people with noise-induced hearing loss have tinnitus. In this case, there is no medical treatment. On the other hand, someone with an acoustic nerve neuroma also may have tinnitus and, in this case, a medical workup is critical. Tinnitus can be an occasional occurrence, or it can be constant. Tinnitus us actually more common than hearing loss, as it believed that over 50 million Americans experience tinnitus to some degree.

Vertigo and Dizziness
True vertigo is a severe spinning sensation usually of short duration. It can be spontaneous, or associated with head movement. The patient can have the sensation the patient spinning themselves or that the

room is spinning around them. There are almost as many causes of dizziness as there are ways in which patients describe it. Recall from Chapter 3, that the balance and auditory system are located in the inner ear Therefore, it is fairly common to encounter patients with hearing loss (especially if it is of relatively of sudden onset) who are also experiencing vertigo.

Otalgia

Simply put, this is ear pain, sometimes called an "earache." Otalgia is not always associated with hearing disorders, as ti can be caused by conditions such as impacted teeth, sinus disease, and inflamed tonsils. If directly related to the ear, it may be due to middle or outer ear pathology.

Aural Fullness

The perceived sensation of a plugged ear that often accompanies vertigo and sudden hearing loss. Aural fullness can also be a symptom of a problem involving the middle ear, often related to poor eustachian tube function.

Hyperacusis

An abnormal sensitivity to sound. Hyperacusis is an internal oveamplification of environmental sounds by the auditory system. Environmental sounds of ordinary intensity that do not bother most people, rally bother those suffering from hyperacusis—e.g., a sound of 65 dB SPL might be perceived like a 100 dB SPL input. This is different from people who simply are "bothered" by loud noise.

Common Hearing Disorders

The most common hearing disorders you will "Encounter" in your daily practice—and some probably will be a mystery. The list is categorized by parts of the ear, and is not an exhaustive list. It is simply a summary of some of the most common conditions, their causes, and audiometric patterns. To make things fairly straightforward, we have organized the disorders as they relate to parts of the ear.

Hearing Disorders of the Outer Ear

Most disorders of the outer ear are easy to observe, respond to treatment, and usually do not cause significant hearing loss. We review five of the most common in this section.

Collapsing Ear Canal

let's talk about an important reason for using them in a little more detail. Some people, especially the elderly, have ear canals that are collapsing. This means that the tissues lining the ear canal have become very soft. This is a normal condition and does not cause hearing loss in the vast majority of cases, because sound only needs a small opening to pass through. But for patients with this problem, this could change when you do a hearing test. When you place supra-aural headphones on someone with collapsing ear canals, it's possible that the pressure will totally collapse the ear canal, and you are actually causing a hearing loss. It is as though the patient is wearing an earplug. This condition results in an audiogram that has the appearance of a conductive hearing loss (usually greatest loss in the higher frequencies, as they are the easiest to attenuate). This easily can be prevented, however, by using inset earphones. Figure 1 gives an example of an audiogram of a patient with collapsing ear canals. The audiogram on the right is after the use of insert phones. note how the loss return to near normal levels (e.g., "correct" values) when the appropriate earphones are used.

Failure to recognize collapsing canals, and the resulting erroneous assumption that there is a conductive hearing loss present, is a good way to lose credibility the physicians that you refer to, as their physical examination clearly will be normal. Of course, if your scope of practice includes the use of immitance audiometry, these results will quickly alert you that the measured air-bone gap is erroneous.

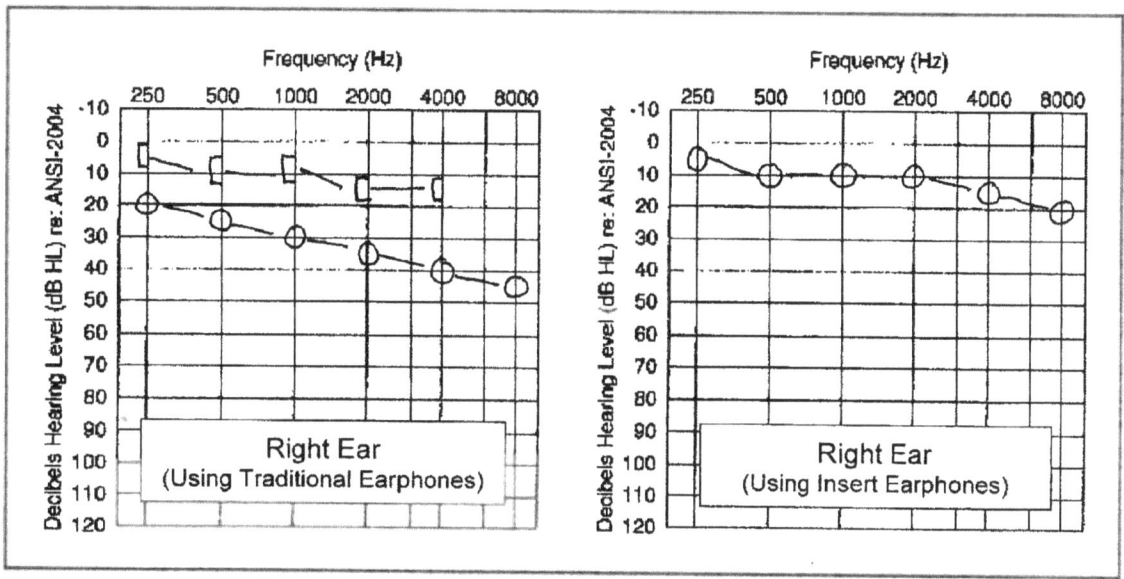

Figure 1 The effects of a collapsing ear canal. The audiogram on the left shows a mild conductive loss when traditional earphones are used. The audiogram on the right shows how air conduction thresholds return to normal levels for the same ear when an insert earphone is used. High frequency conductive losses are rare, so always consider collapsed canals when this pattern is present; the routine use of insert earphones of course will mostly eliminate the problem from the onset.

Impacted Cerumen

Cerumen (or ear wax) is a normal byproduct of a healthy ear. It lubricates the ear canal and protects the canal and tympanic membrane. As cerumen is produced by the subcutaneous glands of the ear canal, it migrates out of the ear canal by way of the tiny hairs lining the outer layer of the external ear canal.

Some people produce more cerument than others, especially the elderly. Additionally, other people may disturb the natural cerumen excretion process by inserting Q-tips and other foreign objects into their ear canal, attempting to remove the cerumen. These objects often irritate the canal, which then results in increased cerumen production, which then results in more probing by the individual, not a good thing. Additionally, using foreign objects to attempt to remove cerumen can result in an impaction, a total blockage of an area of the ear canal.

For individuals who produce excessive cerumen, impaction sometimes also occurs because of hearing aid use. That is, the hearing air (in the case of a custom instrument) or the earmold at the time of each insertion continues to push the cerumen to a given point (usually about 10 to 15 mm from the ear canal opening) and, eventually, a total (or near total) blockage will occur.

Impacted cerumen results in a temporary conductive hearing loss of varying degree (in severe cases, an air-borne gap as large as 30 to 40 dB will be present). Once the cerumen is removed by a qualified professional, hearing returns to pre-impact levels.

External Otitis

Otitis externa is an inflammation of the outer ear and ear canal. Along with otitis media, which we address shortly, external otitis is one of two conditions commonly referred to as an "earache." One common name for this condition is "swimmer's ear" because it frequently develops in people who have been swimming and have had water trapped in their ears.

External otitis is an extremely painful condition requiring treatment from a physician. hearing tests often cannot be conducted on patients with external otitis because the ear is too painful to allow for the placement of earphones.

Acute external otitis often occurs suddenly, rapidly worsens, and becomes extremely painful. Because the tissues lining the external ear canal are extremely thin they are easily torn or abraded by minimal force. Inflammation of the ear canal can begin when someone tried to self-clean their ear canal with a cotton swab or other small implement. Another cause of external otitis is prolonged exposure to water or extreme humidity. Regardless of the cause, external otitis occurs when active bacteria or fungus begin to infect the skin of the ear canal.

Pain that worsens on touching of the outer ear is the predominant complaint associated with external otitis. Patients may also experience discharge from the ear canal and itchiness. Swelling of the ear canal is another symptom and when the swelling is severe enough a conductive hearing loss may occur. In advanced cases of external otitis, pain may radiate to the jaw and neck.

Because the ear is a self-cleaning system, milder cases of this condition can be addressed by simply refraining from swimming or not using implements to try and clear wax from the ear canal. Topical solutions or suspensions in the form of ear drops typically are used to treat mild and moderate cases of otitis externa. In more advanced cases a physician may have to use a binocular microscope to clean the ear canal and insert what is called an ear wick to deliver medication to the infected area.

Tumors of the External Ear Canal

Both malignant and benign tumors have been found in the external ear canal. Bony tumors, called osteomas, are sometimes seen in the ears of people who have done a lot of swimming in cold water. You may not observe a tumor per se, but rather just a narrowing of the canal. Unless the bony growth or tumor closes off the entire external ear canal, they do not cause hearing loss. A detailed ostoscopic exam should reveal this, and, unless this is a long-standing condition reported by the patient, a physician referral is appropriate.

Perforated Tympanic Membrane

There are several ways the tympanic membrane (TM) can become perforated. A perforated eardrum is a rupture of perforation (hole) of the eardrum that can occur as a result of infection, trauma (e.g., by trying to clean the ear with sharp instruments, or even a Q-tip), explosion, barotraumas, or surgery (accidental creation of a rupture).

Because traumatic perforations often alter otherwise normal tissue, they often heal spontaneously. One common cause of TM perforations is related to the buildup of excessive pressure in the middle ear as a result of a middle ear disorder (e.g., eustachian tube dysfunction, infection, effusion, etc.). In these cases, infection, effusion, etc.). In these cases, the excess pressure causes the TM to rupture. Because of the underlying middle ear disorder, TM perforations caused form this excessive pressure need to be managed medically.

Surgical repair of a perforated TM is called myringoplasty or tympanoplasty. In some cases, the "surgical patching" procedures are not successful and the patient more or less will have a "permanent" perforation. Those with more severe and long-standing ruptures may need to wear an earplug to avoid water (or other liquids) making contact with the eardrum, and entering the middle ear cavity.

Perforation of the eardrum usually leads to conductive hearing loss. The amount of hearing loss caused by a perforated TM varies by both the size of the perforation and the location of the opening. Some perforations can be so small that they cannot be detected during routine otoscopy. With large perforations, it's common to see a conductive hearing loss of 30 to 40 dB. Once the perforation heals, hearing is usually recovered fully (maybe with a slight 5- to 10-dB drop due to scarring), but chronic infection over a long period may lead to permanent hearing loss, as the structure of the TM is altered.

Disorders of the Middle Ear

Recall that the purpose of the middle ear is to transmit the airborne sound from the eardrum to the cochlea. This is accomplished quite effectively through the aerial ratio of the TM compared to the oval window, the through the lever action of the ossicular chain. As you would expect, anything that disrupts this flow will cause a middle ear (conductive) hearing loss. We'll describe some of the most common.

Negative Middle Ear Pressure and Middle Ear Effusion

eustachian tube equalizes the pressure between the air filled middle ear and outside air pressure. This tube is normally closed, but when healthy, opens frequently when we talk, chew, yawn, and so forth. When the eustachian tube becomes blocked or swollen from an allergy or common cold, the air pressure outside the middle ear is greater than the air pressure within the middle ear space. Children are more prone to negative middle ear pressure and effusion, because the eustachian tube has not had the opportunity to grow to the proper angle (~45 degrees) and is much more horizontal.

Eustachian tube dysfunction causes the air trapped inside the middle ear to become absorbed by the tissues lining the middle ear space, resulting in a drop in pressure within the middle ear space. The greater pressure from the outside air causes the tympanic membrane to become retracted or pushed into the middle ear space. This condition can be observed with otoscopy, although sometimes it is quite subtle.

A specific audiologic test battery called immittance audiometry is used to measure the function of the entire middle ear system. Tympanometry, which is part of this battery, easily will reveal a retracted TM, or a middle ear system that is not moving effectively.

If negative middle ear pressure continues to develop, and is present for an extended time, the fluids normally secreted by the mucous membranes are collected in the middle ear cavity, resulting in a condition called serous effusion or middle ear effusion. When fluid partially fills the middle ear space a mild to moderate conductive hearing loss can cocur. Often, when a young child has fluid in their middle ears, it is referred to by the lay person (e.g., parents) as an "ear infection." Middle ear effusion, however, is not necessarily infectious.

The audiogram for this patient is directly related to the amount of retraction and/or the amount of fluid in the middle ear. If the patient only has a retracted TM, there probably will be little effect on hearing thresholds. If fluid begins to collect, expect thresholds, especially in the low frequencies, to drop accordingly.

Otitis Media

If middle ear effusion is allowed to continue unabated, otitis media can develop. Otitis media is any infection of the mucous-membrane lining of the middle ear space. Although otitis media is thought of as a disease of childhood, it can occur at any age, and can be quite painful. When these tissues become infected they become swollen, interfering with its pressure equalization function. During this process, the tympanic membrane becomes very vascular, resulting in the TM's red appearance.

There are two types of otitis media, called chronic and acute. As you might imagine, acute otitis media has a very rapid onset time, whereas chronic conditions of otitis media are long-standing. In some cases the fluid in the middle ear becomes thick and sticky and, hence, the nonmedical term "glue ear" sometimes has been used to describe the condition. Like many pathologies of the middle ear, the audiogram will vary with the severity of the problem. It's reasonable to expect a conductive hearing loss of 20 to 30 dB or worse. The configuration might be similar to that shown in Figure 5-2. In severe cases, air-borne gaps of 30 dB or greater are common.

Antibiotics are used in the treatment of otitis media. If otitis media persists, however, pressure equalization (PE) tubes are inserted into the TM by an otolaryngologist. This procedure is called myringotomy with PE tubes. These tubes are also referred to as grommets or tympanostomy tubes. If the tubes are open during audiometric testing (they sometimes become plugged), you would expect to see relatively normal hearing If you conduct immittance testing, volume measures will quickly indicate if the tube is open or closed.

Otosclerosis

Otosclerosis is caused by two main sites of involvement of the sclerotic (or scarlike) lesions. The best understood mechanism is fixation of the stapes footplate to the oval window of the cochlea.

This greatly impairs movement of the stapes and therefore transmission of sound into the inner ear ("ossicular coupling").

Additionalyl, the cochlea's round window can also become sclerotic, and in a similar way impair movement of sound pressure waves through the inner ear ("acoustic coupling"). There is some documentation of sclerotic lesions that also are within the cochlea, sometimes referred to as "cochlear otosclerosis."

Treatment of otosclerosis often involved a surgical procedure called a stapedectomy. A stapedectomy consists of removing a portion of the sclerotic stapes footplate and raplcing it with an implant that is secured to the incus. This procedure restores continuity of ossicular movement and allows transmission of sound waves from the eardrum to the inner ear. A modern variant of this surgery called a stapedotomy, is performed by drilling a small hole in the stapes footplate with a microdrill or a laser, and the insertion of a pistonlike prosthesis.

Otosclerosis can be hereditary, and at least in the early stages, results in a conductive hearing loss of mild to modereate-severe degree, usually with the greatest loss in the lower frequencies. In the later stages, a mixed hearing loss may be present. Figure 2 gives an example of otosclerosis you might see in your office or on an audiogram. While this patient certainly is a hearing aid candidate, and probably would be a successful user of hearing aids, most opt for surgical treatment. Typically, following surgery there is a significant improvement in air conduction thresholds.

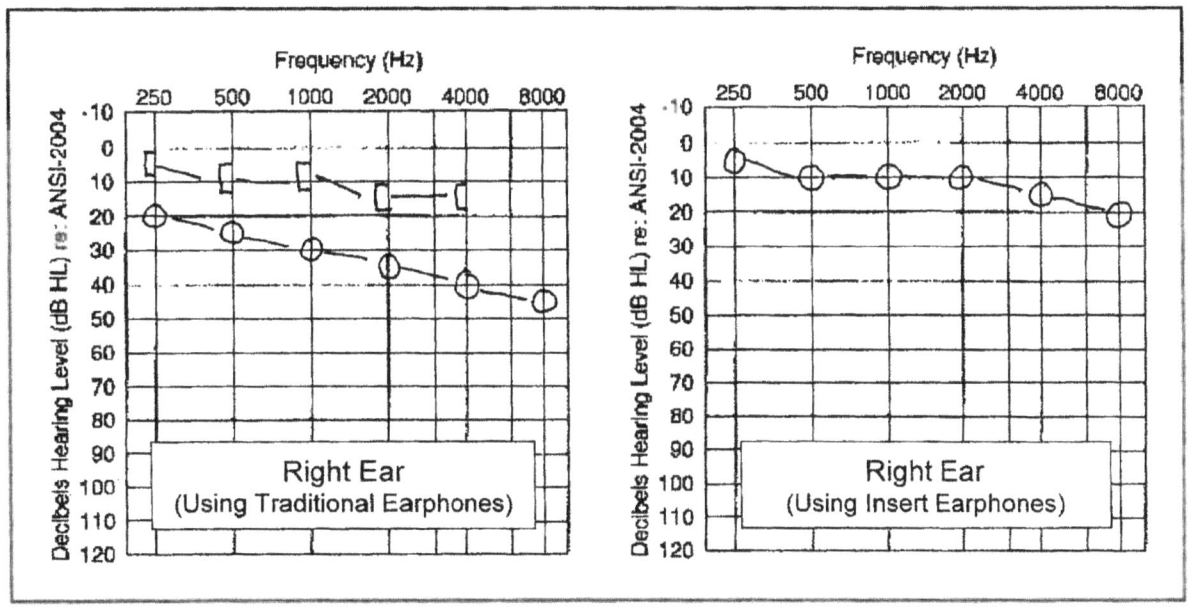

Figure 2. A bilateral conductive hearing loss consistent with bilateral otosclerosis. Notice the 2000 Hz or "Carhart" notch in the bone conduction scores in both ears.

Cholesteatoma

In general, cholesteatomas are the result of a long-standing middle ear condition. Cholesteatomas from a sac with concentric rings consisting of a protein called keratin; there is some evidence to classify them as low-grade tumors. In patients with TM perforations, the tissue may enter the middle ear through the perforation, producing a cholesteatoma. Cholesteatomas may also be caused by chronic episodes of otitis media. Cholesteatomas are dangerous because they eventually can erodes the bones of the middle ear. They potentially also could damage the facial nerve, and will even invade the nose and brain cavity in rare instances. In most cases cholesteatoma are removed with surgery. As with other middle ear pathologies, the patient will have a conductive hearing loss, although the patient with a cholesteatoma will typically have a more severe loss than most other middle ear conditions, due to the extent of the disease. It's common to observe air-bone gaps of 30 to 40 dB. A sample case study is shown in Figure 3.

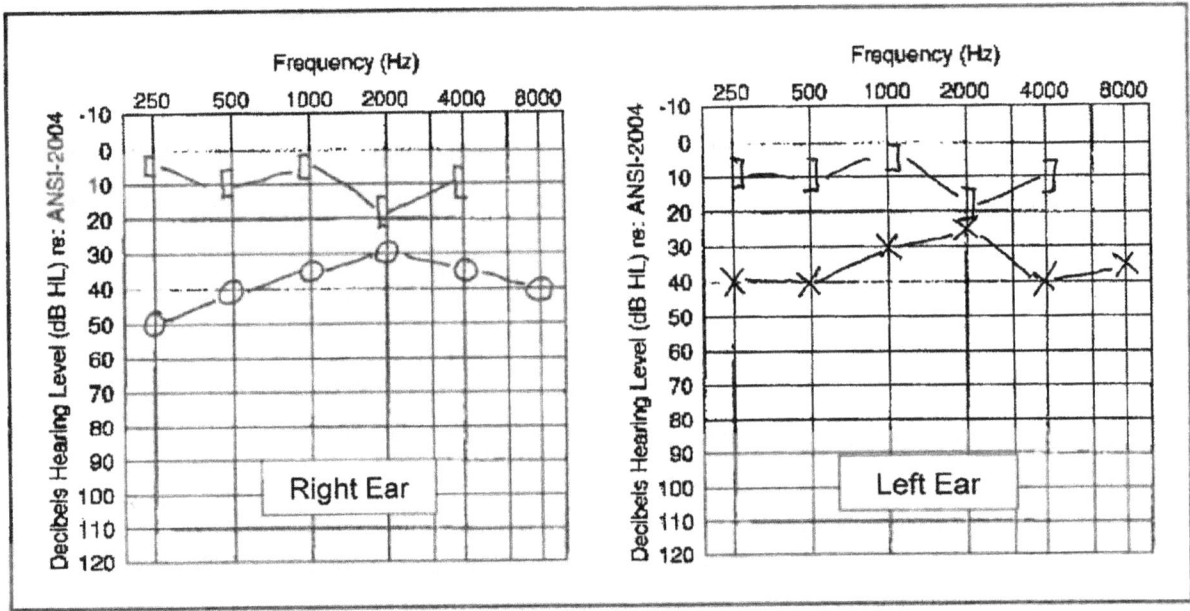

Figure 3. A bilateral conductive hearing loss associated with a cholesteatoma in the right ear, and otitis media in the left.

Tympanosclerosis
Tympanosclerosis is characterized by white plaques on the surface of the tempanic membrane and deposits on the ossicles. It is often the result of chronic otitis media, which when untreated leaves this white residue. Tympanosclerosis can have a stiffening effect on the TM, which may result in a conductive hearing loss in the low frequencies. As mention earlier, PE tubes are a common treatment for otitis media. It's common for these patients (~30 to 40%) to have resulting tympanosclerosis after the tubes have fallen out, or been removed.

Ossicular Disarticulation
This is also referred to as "dislocation" or "discontinuity." As the name indicates, this condition results in one of the two joints between the three ossicles being pulled apart or disarticulated (the incudostapedial juncture is the most common). It can produce a wide variety of conductive hearing losses depending on the location and extent of the disarticulation. The most common causes of ossicular

disarticulation are degenerative diseases and trauma to the head. In severe head trauma a TM perforation also might be observed. Interestingly, the largest hearing loss (conductive) is present when the TM is intact, not perforated. In these cases, it is possible for an ossicular disarticulation to cause up to a 50 to 60 dB conductive hearing loss, as the cochlea is stimulated via bone conduction for higher levels (see Figure 3).

Patulous Eustachian Tube

In some cases the eustachian tube, which is ordinarily closed, is chronically open (patent). These persons often complain that their own voices sound hollow or that they hear their own breathing inside their head. Many of these patients have an overly patent or patulous eustachian tube. One of the more common reasons for having a patulous esutachian tube is a loss of a significant amount of weight. Although a patulous eustachian tube is not a pathologic condition, it can be quite annoying. Immitance audiometry which we briefly mentioned in Chapter can be used to identify patulous eustachian tubes. There is little or no accompanying hearing loss.

Disorders of the Cochlea

A significant number of people around the world have sensorineural hearing loss as a consequence of damage to the cochlea. For adults, sensorineural hearing loss resulting from cochlear pathology is by far the most common type of hearing impairment. In this section we spend some time reviewing the most common types of sensorineural hearing loss resulting from cochlear pathology. Because there is very limited medical or surgical treatment of cochlear hearing loss, these are the people that you will likely see for hearing aid fitting.

Presbycusis

If your patient is beyond the age of 60 years old, it's possible that the hearing sensitivity has progressively worsened over the years, and this will now be reflected in the audiogram, especially in the higher frequencies. This gradual deterioration of hearing is often a result of presbycusis (sometimes written "presbyacusis"). Simply stated, presbycusis is hearing loss caused by the cumulative effects of the aging process. This progression is somewhat more rapid for men than for women, although this partially could be due to the fact that men experience more noise exposure than women, which is difficult to separate from the aging effects on the inner ear structures.

Presbycusis affects all parts of the ear, including neural transmissions to the brain, but the primary site of lesion is the cochlea. The outer hair cells within the cochlea are particularly sensitive to the wear and tear associated with the aging process. As a general rule, the higher the frequency, the greater effect of presbycusis (even people in their 20s and 30s experience loss of sensitivity in the >16,000-Hz range).

The classic presbycusis audiogram will show a gradually sloping downward pattern; nearly always, as the frequency becomes higher the hearing loss becomes worse (Figure 4).

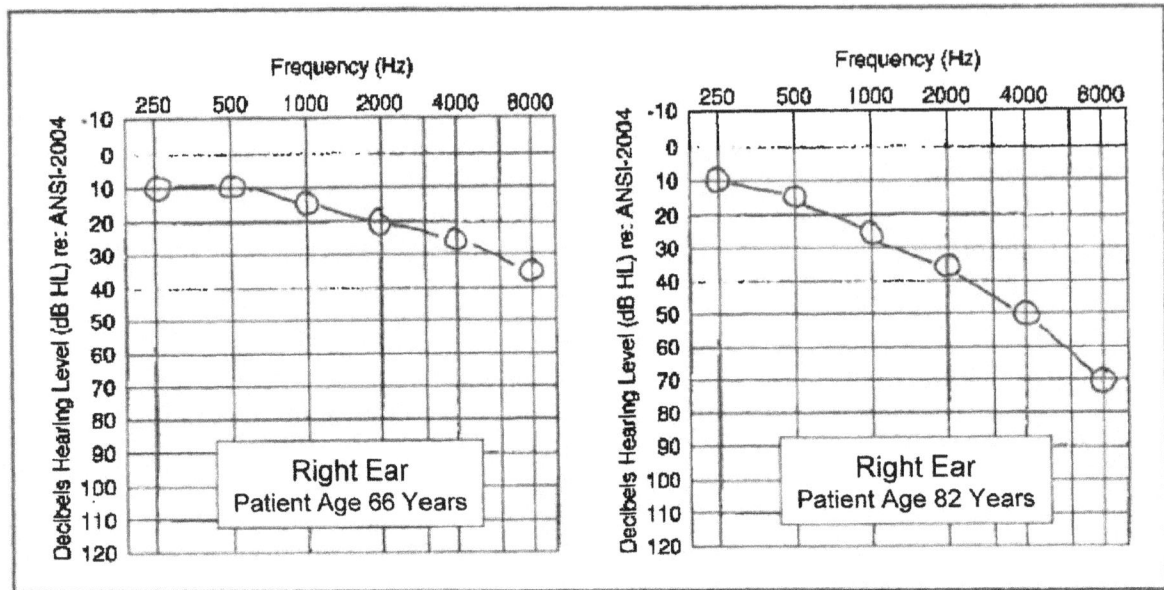

Figure 4. The progressive nature of presbycusis for an individual's left ear. The audiogram on the left is from a 66-year-old male (showing a slight noise notch with some recovery at 8000 Hz; given the relatively good threshold at 8000 Hz we would predict that presbycusic effects are minimal at this time). The audiogram on the right is for the same male patient at the age of 82. Note that the pattern now no longer looks like a noise-induced hearing loss, as the high-frequency presbycusis effects have bended into the previous 800- to 4000-Hz hearing loss. We only show the left ear thresholds, but typically a symmetrical pattern is observed.

Noise-Induced Hearing Loss (NIHL)

Exposure to loud sounds can result in temporary or permanent hearing loss. This condition is called noise-induced hearing loss (NIHL).

Around 30 million adults in the United States are exposed to hazardous sound levels in the workplace. Among there 30 million people, it's estimated that one in four will acquire a permanent hearing loss as a result of their occupation.

The degree of hearing loss caused by NIHL depends on the intensity of the sound, duration of the exposure, frequency spectrum of the sound, individual susceptibility, along with other variables. Usually this type of hearing loss is due to continued exposure to work or recreational noise exposure that has occurred over several years. It is possible, however, for NIHL to occur for only a very short duration of exposure, or even a single blast (Referred to as "acoustic trauma"). Because of the shape of the cochlea and the resonant effects of the outer ear, most cases of NIHL show a high-frequency hearing loss, with maximum loss in the 3000 to 6000-Hz range, and usually with some recovery at the highest frequencies. This pattern on the audiogram is called a "noise notch" (see Figure 5-5). NIHL can affect people of all ages.

As NIHL is a fairly common condition it is worth spending a little bit of time discussing the reason for the precipitous slope and noise notch. There are a couple of reasons why the area around

4000 KHz is most susceptible to damage. Although the noise causing NIHL may be broadband, with roughly equal amplitude at all frequencies, the outer ear and ear canal resonances have amplified the noise in the 2000 to 4000-kHZ region by the time the sound reaches the cochlea. This region, therefore, shows the greatest amount of damage from noise exposure. Another reason for NIHL causing more loss in the high frequencies compared to the lows is related to cochlear mechanics and cochlear blood flow; the positioning of the 3000 to 4000-Hz hair cell receptors along the basal turn of the cochlea. It is possible, but quite uncommon, for a noise notch to occur at lower frequencies (e.g., 500 to 1500 Hz; this is most commonly observed when the person was continuously exposed to a unique noise of a narrow bandwidth.

No matter the underlying reason NIHL is a common etiology of cochlear pathology. Given its prevalence, patients that are exposed to both workplace and recreational noise need to be using properly fitted hearing protection. Counseling regarding the need for hearing protection is part of all audiologic exams.

NIHL in its most common form is of gradual onset. The two audiograms below are from the same factory worker taken 8 years apart. Notice that the loss has become worse over the 10 year period. People with significant NIHL routinely are fitted with hearing aids, however, because many with NIHL have normal hearing for low-frequency sounds they sometimes are challenging to fit. Many people with the hearing loss shown in the audiogram shown in Figure-5 say they can *hear*, but they just can't *understand* completely. This is due to the normal low-frequency hearing, which provides them "loudness," but the missing high frequencies reduces the audibility of critical speech cues for understanding.

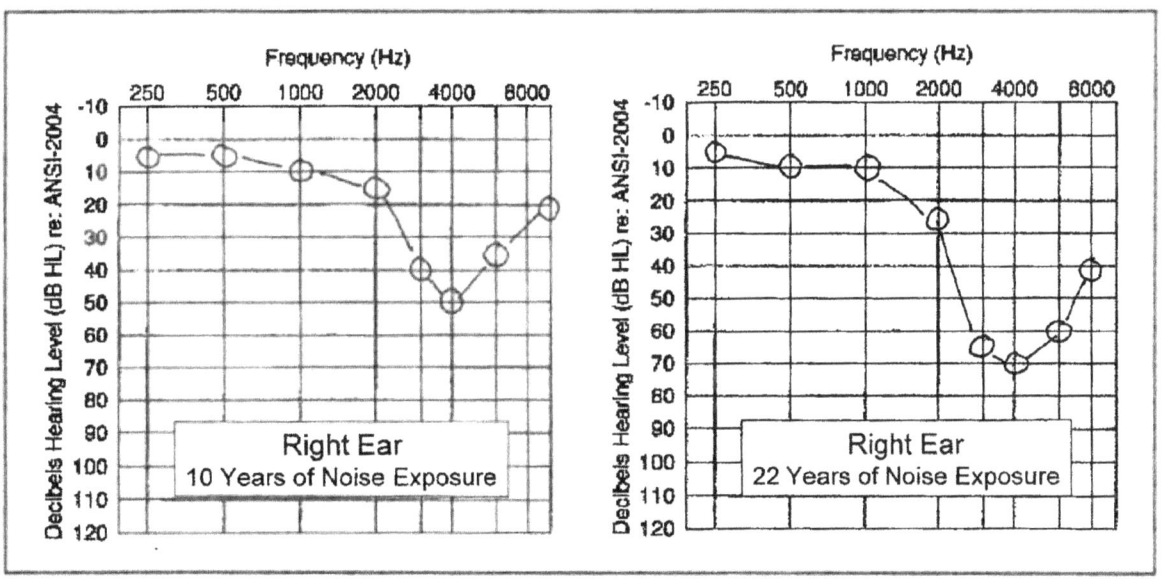

Figure 5. The effects of NIHL over time for one individual's left ear. Thresholds were measured 12 years apart for a male patient working in a condition of intense noise (daily carpentry with skill saw). The audiogram on the right shows the progressive nature of the hearing loss consistent with the patient's history of noise exposure. Notice how the dip at 400 Hz deepens, and other frequencies become more involved. The left ear had the same pattern but was not as severe; perhaps there was some attenuation of the noise from head shadow for this ear.

Permissible Levels

Our review of noise-induce hearing loss would not be complete without a discussion of permissible levels of noise exposure. There is a direct relationship between the intensity of noise, the duration of the exposure, and the degree of potential NIHL. When counseling patients about noise exposure, it's good to have a general idea of what is "safe," and when hearing protection is needed. The Occupational Health and Safety Agency (OSHA) is an arm of the federal government responsible for ensuring that workers are safely protected from dangerous amounts of noise. Table 4-1 indicates when the intensity and duration of exposure becomes dangerous for individuals. If a worker is exposed to levels of sounds greater than 90 dB for 8 hours per day, they are required to wear hearing protection. Notice that as the intensity increases the exposure time needed to cause damage is reduced.

90 dB	8.0 hours
92 dB	6.0 hours
95 dB	4.0 hours
97 dB	3.0 hours
100 dB	2.0 hours
102 dB	1.5 hours
105 dB	1.0 hours
110 dB	30 minutes
115 dB	15 minutes

Table 4-1. Maximum Permissible Noise Levels
Source: Downloaded from http://www.quietsolution.com/Noise_Levels.pdf

Viral and Bacterial Diseases

There are several viral and bacterial infections that can result in sensorineural hearing loss. Infections, such as cytomegalovirus, can be transmitted to the child from the mother in utero. This is a condition known as prenatal. The following diseases are considered prenatal conditions that can result in a congenital hearing loss:

- Syphilis
- Rubella
- Toxoplasmosis
- Cytomegalovirus (CMV)
- Herpes simplex virus

There also are several viral and bacterial infections that occur after a child has been born that can produce sensorineural hearing loss. In most cases these postnatal infections enter the inner ear through the blood supply, which is carrying the infection. The following are some of the most common diseases acquired after birth (postnatal) causing hearing loss:

- Mumps
- Measles
- Bacterial meningitis

It may be obvious to some, but workplaces are not the only conditions causing NIHL. there are plenty of recreational activities, like hunting, drag racing, and going to the disco that can caus NIHL/ Even though OSHA's Permissible Noise Exposure chart wasn't created with them in mind, if you have a sound level meter, you can determine if your nightclub activities are causing some permanent hearing loss.

Ototoxicity

There are several drugs used for therapeutic treatment of diseases that have the potential side effect of causing damage to the inner ear. Because the cochlea is such a delicate organ it is susceptible to damage from medications and chemical agents. Such drugs and agents are considered to be ototoxic or poisonous to the ears.

Ototoxic drugs have one thing in common: they cause a sensorineural hearing loss. The amount of ototoxic hearing loss depends on the exact dosage and duration of use. When you encounter a patient who has used or been exposed to an ototoxic medication or agent you should consult a physician or pharmacist. A ototoxic hearing loss can present itself in different ways, but, typically, the high frequencies are the first affected, and the hearing loss is usually downward sloping. Some facilities conduct high-frequency audiometry (10,000 to 18,000 Hz) to monitor early changes in hearing.

There are hundreds of otoxic medications and agents. The most common ones along with their therapeutic uses are listed in Table 5-1. Also listed is whether the drug causes a permanent or reversible hearing loss. The majority of drugs cause a permanent hearing loss.

Type of Drug	Type of Hearing Loss	Reversible? (Y/N)
1. **Aminoglycoside Antibiotics** • streptomycin • gentamycin • kanamycin • vancomycin	Sensorineural	No
2. **Cancer Chemotherapeutics** • cisplatin • carboplatin	Sensorineural	No
3. **Loop Diuretics (Furosemide)** • lasix • bumax	Sensorineural	Yes
4. **Salicylates** • aspirin	Sensorineural	Yes
5. **Quinine**	Sensorineural	Yes

Table 4-2. A Summary of Common Drug Types and Their Effects on Hearing

This list is by no means exhaustive; rather, it is designed to represent a sample of the most common ototoxic agents you will encounter. Because new medications are always being introduced onto the market it is best to consult with your local physician or pharmacist for the most current information.

Ototoxic hearing loss is relatively common in patients receiving platinum-based chemotherapy drugs. According to several studies between 23 and 61% developed sensorineural hearing loss as a result of receiving these chemotherapy drugs. In many cases these hearing losses develop 100 to 135 days following the onset of the chemotherapy regiment. Some of the more common platinum-based agents include cisplatin, carboplatin, eloxtin, and vincristine.

Figure 6 shows two audiograms form a patient who has been receiving large doses of ciplatin for lung cancer. the first audiogram is 1 month after the first treatment and the second audiogram is 60 days later. Note the difference in the thresholds due to the treatment duration. As a dispensing professional you probably will not be directly involved in collecting these types of serial audiograms; however, it's important to note how and when various treatments may affect someone' shearing and associated hearing aid use.

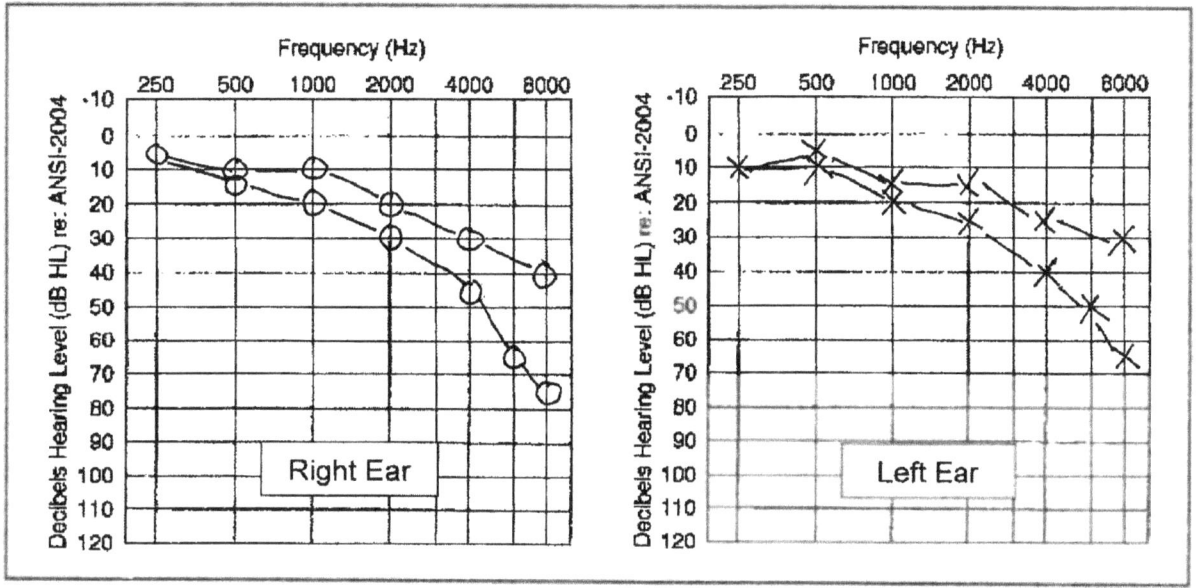

Figure 6. Audiograms for a patient taking larges doses of cisplatin. The upper (better) is 30 days after the first treatment and the lower (worse) audiogram on the right is 60 days after the first treatment. Note the decline in hearing over that period of time, which can be attributed to the drug regimen. The bilateral downward-sloping pattern is common.

Ménière's Disease

Ménière's disease is name after the French physician Prosper Ménière, who first reported that vertigo was caused by inner ear disorders in an article published in 1861. Ménière's disease, in its "classic form" is used to describe a hearing disorder with one or more of the following characteristics:

1   A hearing loss (usually in one ear) of sudden or rapid onset.
2   A fullness or pressure sensation in the ear.
3   Brief and sudden episodes of severe dizziness (vertigo)
4   A roaring (tinnitus) in the affected ear.

One or all of the symptoms require an immediate referral to a physician. There are many subcategories of Ménière's disease beyond the scope of this chapter. Some types of cochlear hearing losses of sudden onset, such as Ménière's, although they are sensorineural many cases actually return to normal levels.

The exact cause of Ménière's disease is not known, but it is believed to be related to *endolymphatic hydrops* or excess fluid in the inner ear. It is thought that endolymphatic fluid bursts from its normal channels in the ear and flows into other areas causing damage. this is called "hydrops." This may be related to swelling of the endolymphatic sac or other tissues in the vestibular system of the inner ear, which is responsible for the body's sense of balance.

There is no standard "signature" audiogram for Ménière's, but in general there tends to be more low-frequency hearing loss than observed for most other sensorineural pathologies. That is, the audiogram often appears "flat" or upward sloping rather than the more common downward sloping pattern. Figure 7 shows an audiogram of a client diagnosed with Ménière's disease. Not the asymmetric (unilateral) nature of the hearing loss. After this hearing loss has stabilized, and the physician has given authorization, this person might be fit with a hearing aid in the affected ear.

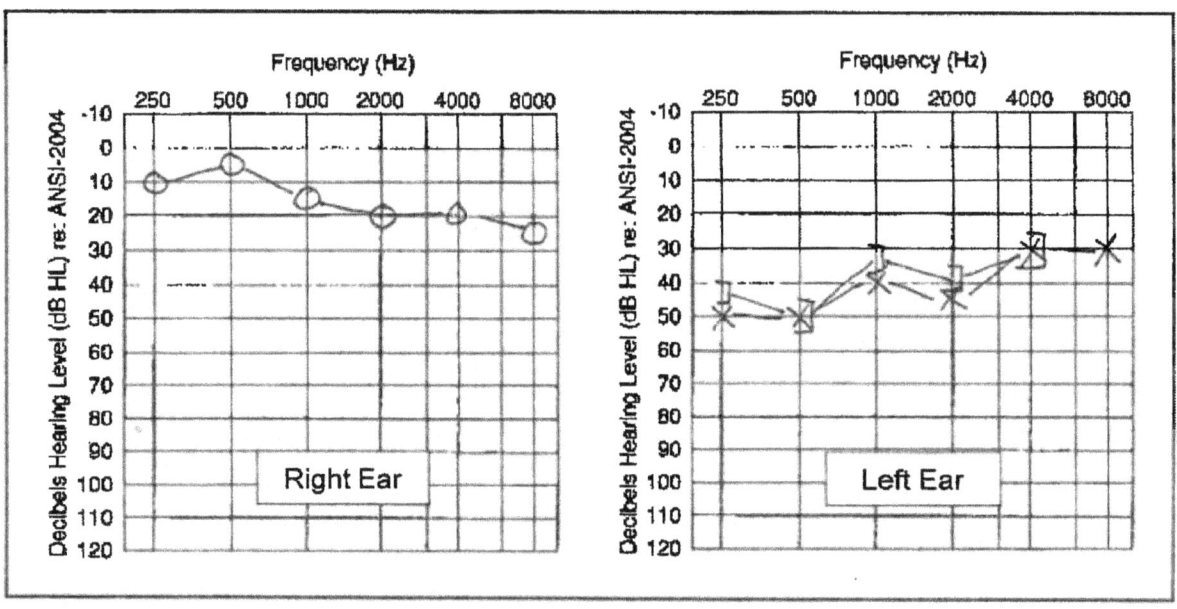

Figure 7. Asymmetric left sensorineural hearing loss consistent with Ménière's disease.

Retrocochlear Disorders

In general terms, retrocochlear disorders or pathology refers to damage to the nerve fibers along the ascending auditory pathways, running from the internal auditory canal to the auditory cortex. In other words, we might be quite certain that the problem does not lie within the middle ear or the cochlea, and therefore, the locus must be somewhere more medial. Commonly, in audiologic practice, retrocochlear is used to refer to the eighth nerve and the low brainstem, and the auditory dysfunction at higher auditory levels is referred to as "central."

In most cases, eighth nerve retrocochlear pathologies involved tumors. Retrocochlear tumors, referred to as acoustic schmannomas, acoustic neuromas, neurinomas, or neurilemomas, typically (but not always) produce unilateral high-frequency hearing loss in their more advanced stages. And, unlike presbycusis and many other types of *cochlear* pathology, it is unlikely that there would be uniform symmetric tumors, so there usually is asymmetry between ears in the audiogram (Figure-8.)

The signs and symptoms of eighth nerve retrocochlear pathology are subtle and difficult to identify with conventional audiometry. In many cases, in the early stages, there is no significant hearing loss (although there may be a reduction of speech understanding for speech in noise, or other difficult speech tests). Many patients will complain of tinnitus on the affected side, vertigo or dizziness, fullness, or speech not sounding clear. In cases where retrocochlear pathology is suspected, a complete audiologic diagnostic battery and otologic referral is needed. Your job is to refer the patient to a physician or audiologist if a "red flag" for a retrocochlear pathology exists.

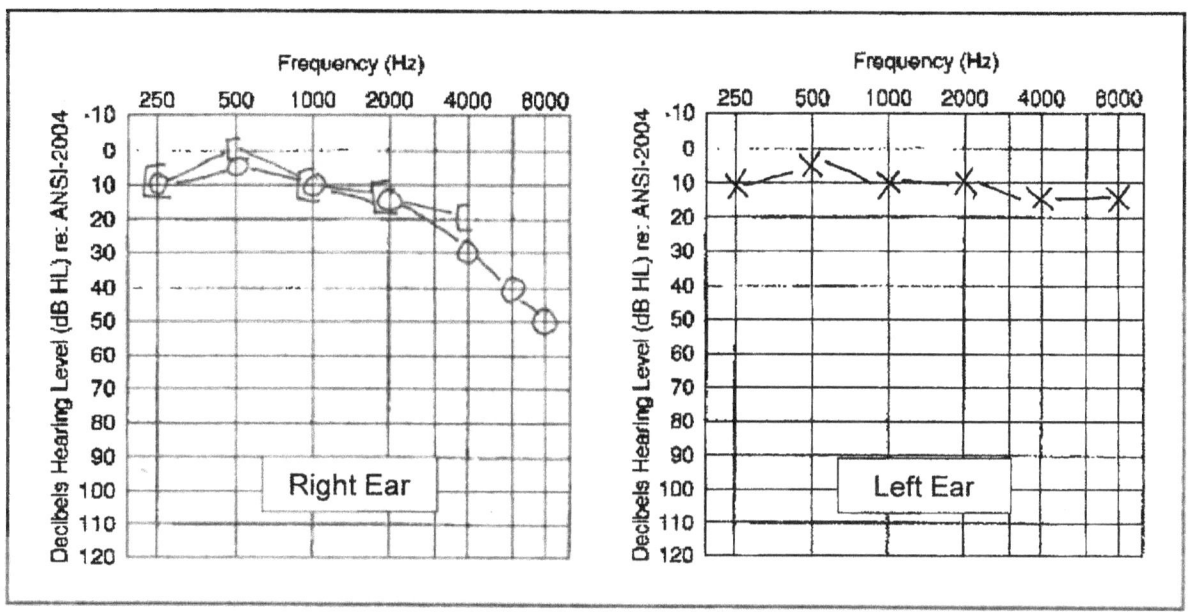

Figure 8. A mild, right asymmetric sensorineural hearing loss consistent with possible retrocochlear pathology.

Central Auditory Disorders

As mentioned earlier, technically a retrocochlear patholofy would include everything medial of the cochlea, but usually we refer to pathology above the low brainstem as "Central." When thinking about auditory disorders, it's important to remember the "Subtlety principle." That is, as the pathology becomes more central, going from the middle ear to the auditory cortex, the impact of the disorder on traditional audiologic tests will be more subtle. For example, a cochlear pathology will nearly always cause a reduction in hearing thresholds and speech understanding. A disorder of the brainstem (e.g., multiple sclerosis, tumors, etc.) may cause no hearing loss and no loss of speech understanding (unless a difficult speech-in-noise test is conducted).

Nonorganic Hearing Loss

There may be cases where a hearing loss may be measured on the audiogram, but there is no organic basis to explain the impairment. Some of the terms used to describe this include nonorganic hearing loss, pseudohypocusis, and functional hearing loss. If indeed the patient knowingly is exaggerating their hearing loss, the term malingering is used.

Aside from the cases of malingering, where with adults, exaggeration of the hearing loss usually is related to financial compensation, the reasons for nonorganic hearing loss are not clearly understood. A number of signs can alert you to the possibility, however. These signs may include inconsistent test results, poor test-retest reliability, inappropriate behavior during the test (e.g., exaggerated attempt at listening or lipreading), or poor agreement between test results and real-world communication (e.g., the patient answers your questions in the waiting room, but then demonstrates a flat 70 dB HL hearing loss). Is some cases, there may be an underlying hearing loss, and the patient is simply adding to it.

One reason SRTs should be conducted during routine testing is to cross check the reliability of pure-tone thresholds. If the SRT and pure-tone average differ by more than 10 dB, the reliability of the test should be questioned. If there is a discrepancy, the SRT will nearly always be *better than* the pure-tone average. We recommend conducting the SRT before the pure-tone thresholds, as this will provide you with a general idea of where the thresholds should be falling for the speech frequencies, as you would simply assume that the entire exam is invalid. Many other special tests have been developed to detect nonorganic hearing loss, including the Stenger test which is very effective when the loss is only in one ear.

Other rare unusual causes of conductive hearing loss are Malleus fixation, Cerebral spinal fluid leak, third window lesions, Paget bone disease, Superior Semicircular Canal Dehiscence (SSCD), Aberrant Carotid Canal, and X-linked Hearing Loss. The Malleus fixation is in the middle ear and the rest are inner ear lesions.

Malleus Fixation is calcification of the supporting ligament of the superior malleus and it occurs at later in life. The symptoms mimic Otosclerosis. See chart below to see how they differentiate.

Otosclerosis	Malleus Fixation
Air bone gap: 0-60 dB in all freq.	0-60 dB low freq.
BC thresholds: < 0 dB	< 0 dB
Acoustic Reflexes: absent	present/absent
Involve Ears: bilateral	unilateral
Age of presentation: Teen/adult	later decades
HL progression: gradual	gradual
Pneumo-Otoscopy: Malleus mobile,	Malleus immobile
Ossicular Chain: Fixed or discontinuity	normal
CT Scan: Otosclerotic foci	normal

Rare Hearing Losses and Causes

Abnormal inner ear function occurs in the present of a Scala Vestibuli: X-linked Hearing loss, large vestibular Aqueduct and Aberrant Carotid Canal dehiscence and finally a Superior Semicircular Canal Dehiscence. Energy is they deviated from the Cochlea producing a Conductive Hearing loss in the inner ear.

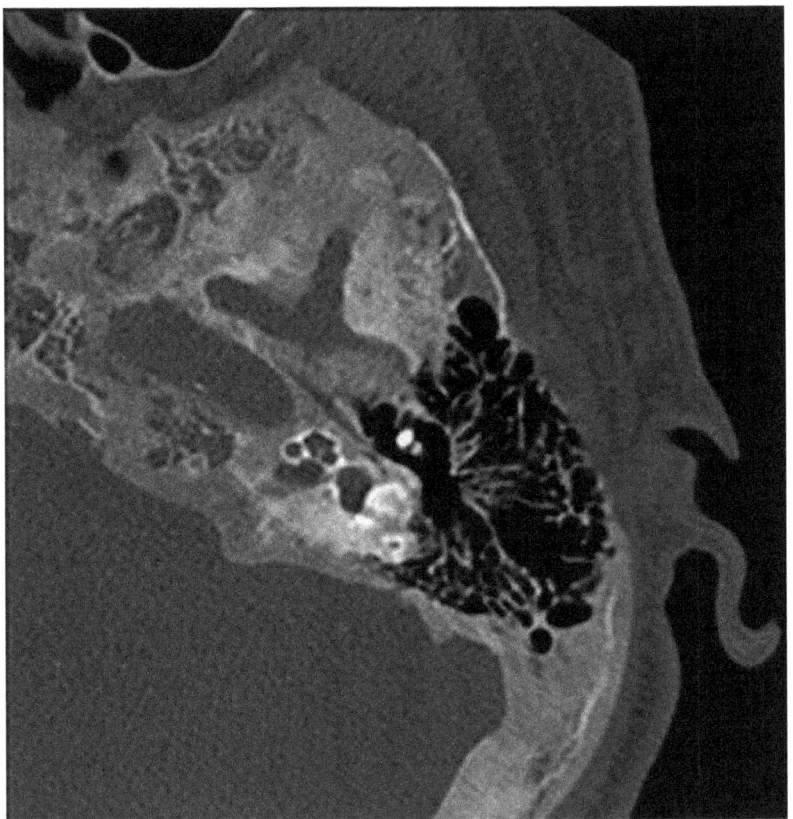

Paget's Disease

The Malleus Fixation differentiates form the 3rd Window and SCCD. See chart below to see how they differentiate.

MF	**3rd Window**
AB gap: 0-60 dB low-mid freq.	0-60 dB <2 kHz
BC Thresholds: < 0 dB	-5 to -20 dB <2 kHz
Acoustic Reflexes: absent	present
Tympanometry: Type B	Type A
OAE: absent	present
VEMPs absent	present
Loud noise dizziness: absent	present
Ossicular Chain: Fixed	normal
CT scan: Calcified malleus ligaments	normal

Superior Canal Dehiscence Syndrome

Superior canal dehiscence syndrome (SCDS) is a rare medical condition of the inner ear, leading to hearing and balance symptoms in those affected. The symptoms are caused by a thinning or complete absence of the part of the temporal bone overlying the superior semicircular canal of the vestibular system. There is evidence that this rare defect, or susceptibility, is congenital.

Dizziness/vertigo/chronic disequilibrium caused by the dysfunction of the superior semicircular canal, Tullio phenomenon (sound-induced vertigo), disequilibrium or dizziness, nystagmus and oscillopsia, Pulse-synchronous oscillopsia, Hyperacusis (the over sensitivity to sound), Low frequency conductive hearing loss, A feeling of fullness in the affected ear, Pulsatile tinnitus, Brain fog Fatigue, Headache/migraine, Tinnitus (high-pitched ringing in the ear). The audiogram would demonstrate mixed hearing loss at with high frequency conductive hearing loss and the least conductive hearing loss would be at 2 KHz. The speech discrimination would be good, acoustic reflexes would be absent on the affected ear, the tympanogram would be Type A, absent OAE, positive VEMP, Abnormal ABR, and VNG would show unilateral Vertigo. Spiral 1 mm cuts CAT scan would show a dehiscence of the superior Semicircular Canal.

Symptoms of SCDS include: Autophony (person's own speech) or other self-generated noises (e.g. heartbeat, eye movements, and creaking joints, chewing) are heard unusually loudly in the affected ear.

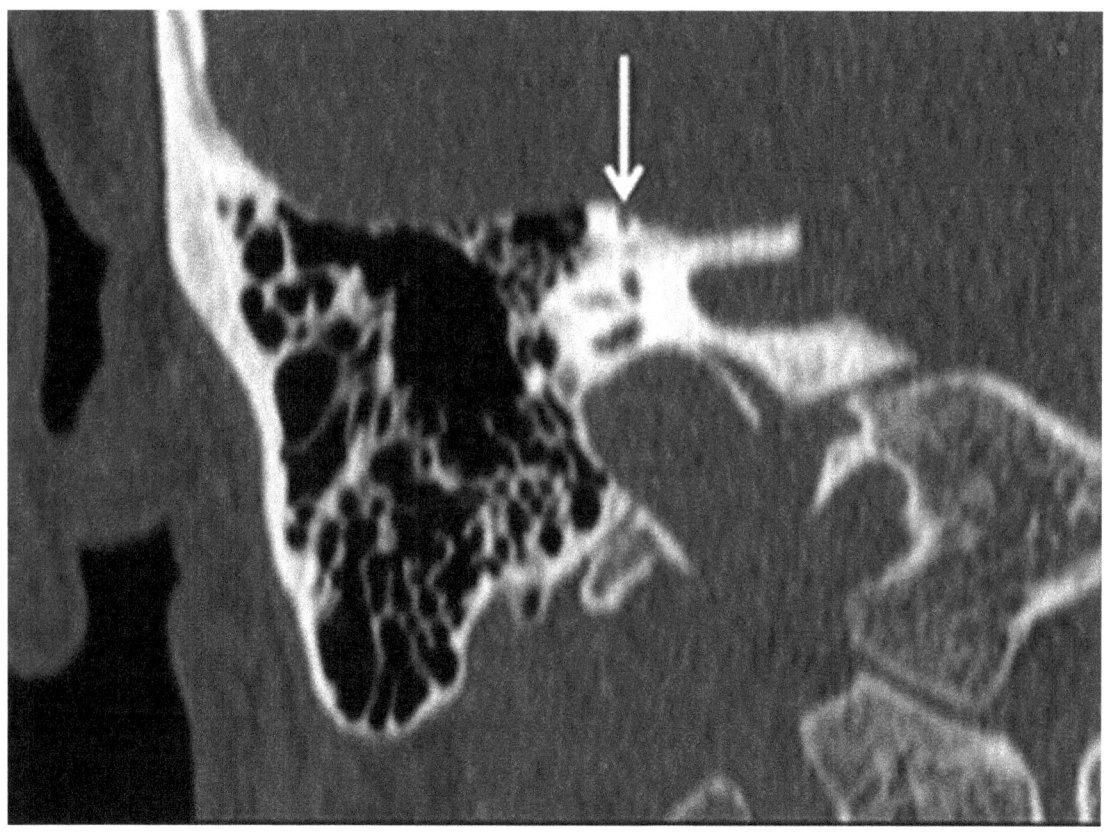

Superior Semicircular Canal Dehiscence (SSCD)

Large Vestibular Aqueduct Syndrome

Large vestibular aqueduct syndrome (LVAS) refers to the presence of congenital sensorineural hearing loss with an enlarged vestibular aqueduct. It is thought to be one of the most common congenital causes of sensorineural hearing loss (SNHL). The vestibular aqueduct acts as a canal between the inner ear and the cranial cavity. Running through it is a tube called the endolymphatic duct, which normally carries a fluid called endolymph from the inner ear to the endolymphatic sac in the cranial cavity. When the endolymphatic duct and sac are larger than normal, as is the case in large vestibular aqueduct syndrome, endolymph is allowed to travel back from the endolymphatic sac into the inner ear. This often results from abnormal or delayed development of the inner ear during childhood. Enlarged vestibular aqueduct syndrome is often comorbid with other inner ear development problems, such as cochlear deformities. Studies show that genetic defects such as Pendred syndrome are related to large vestibular aqueduct syndrome, and have connected the disorder specifically to a defect on chromosome 7q31.

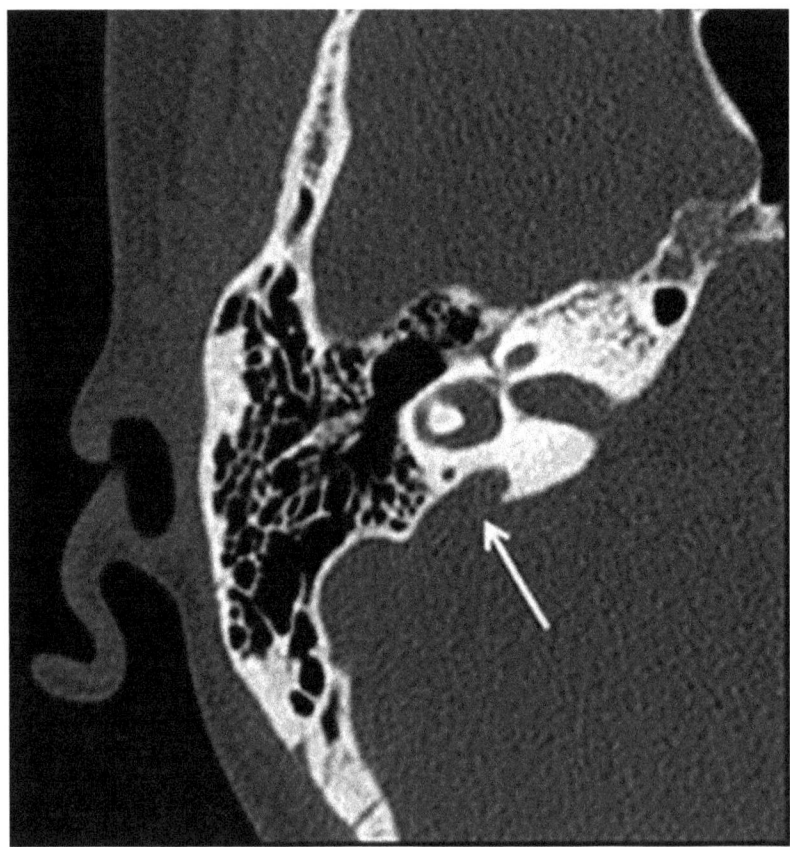

Vestibular Aqueduct

The audiogram would demonstrate a severe to profound SNHL, poor discrimination, absent acoustic reflexes, absent OAE, Type A tympanogram, Abnormal ABR and VNG/vHIT wound demonstrate a unilateral Vertigo. CAT scan would demonstrate a large vestibular aqueduct with normal SCC. VEMP would be normal.

Auditory Neuropathy Spectrum Disorder

Auditory Neuropathy Spectrum Disorder (ANSD) is a specific form of hearing loss defined by the presence of normal or near-normal Otoacoustic Emissions (OAEs) but the absence of normal middle ear reflexes and severely abnormal or completely absent auditory brainstem response (ABRs). This is cause by the lack of the transmission of sound from the inner ear to the brain. The cause is believed to be from birth complications and genetics.

Audiogram would demonstrate various thresholds; however, according to Dr. Hall, low-frequency hearing loss is the most common, in addition to poor speech discrimination score as compared to the hearing loss, absent acoustic reflexes, normal OAE with absent ABR. Type A tympanograms. Normal CT of brain.

Normal Inner Ear Function

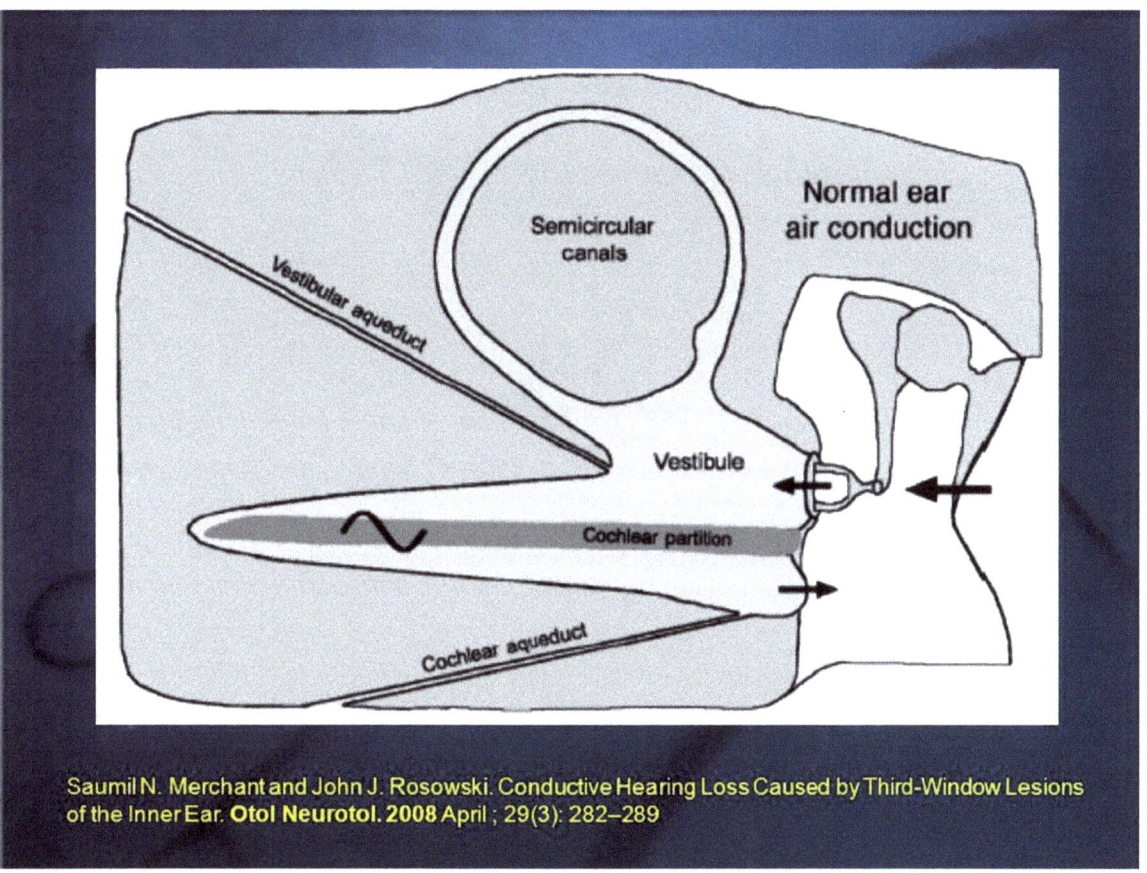

Saumil N. Merchant and John J. Rosowski. Conductive Hearing Loss Caused by Third-Window Lesions of the Inner Ear. **Otol Neurotol. 2008** April ; 29(3): 282–289

Energy from sound inters the inner ear via the oval window and the energy is distributed from the oval window cochlear portion of the inner ear.

Abnormal Inner Ear Function

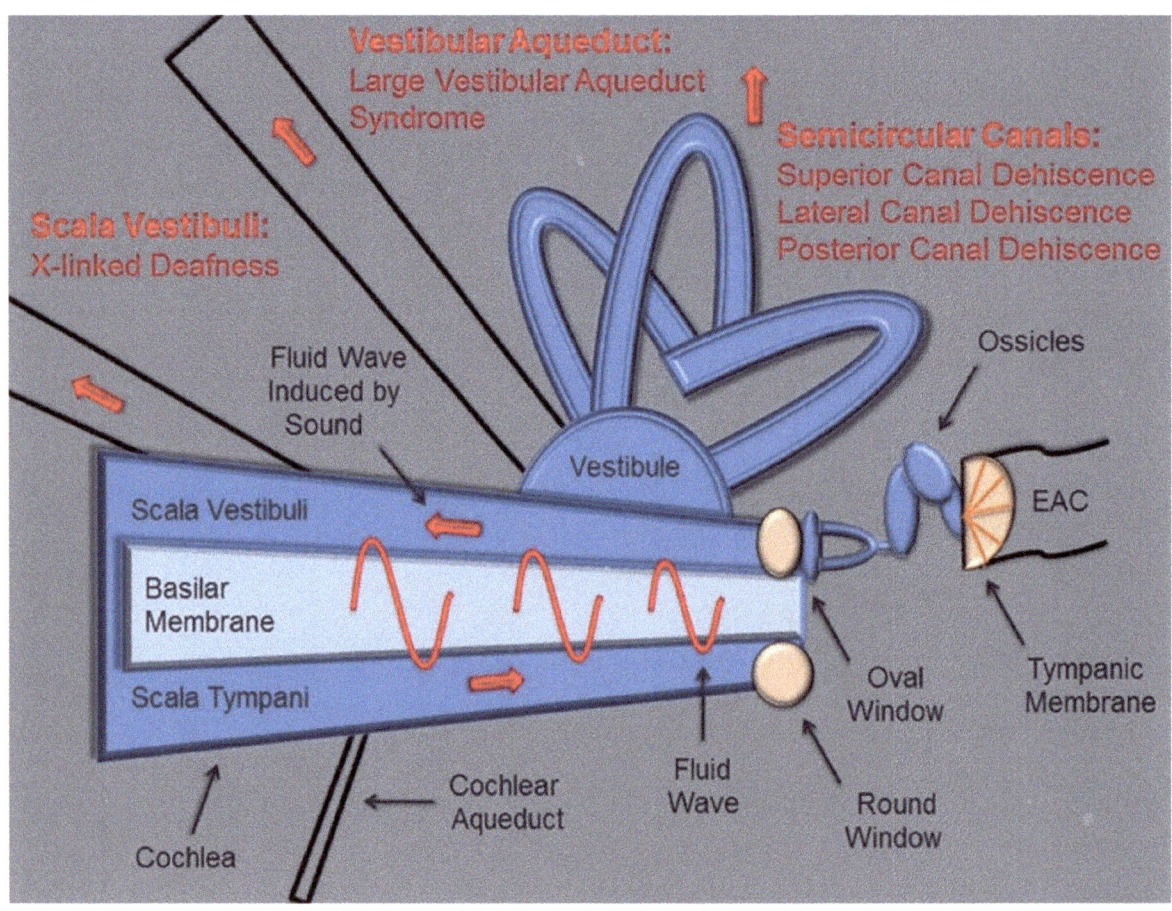

Sara J. Moren MD, Msci: Alexander W. Korutz, MD, Achilles G. Karagranis DO, Courtney CJ Voelker, MD, PhD, Alexander J Nemeth, MD.

The following are samples of the CT finding in all the Inner Ear lesions:

X linked Hearing Loss Syndrome

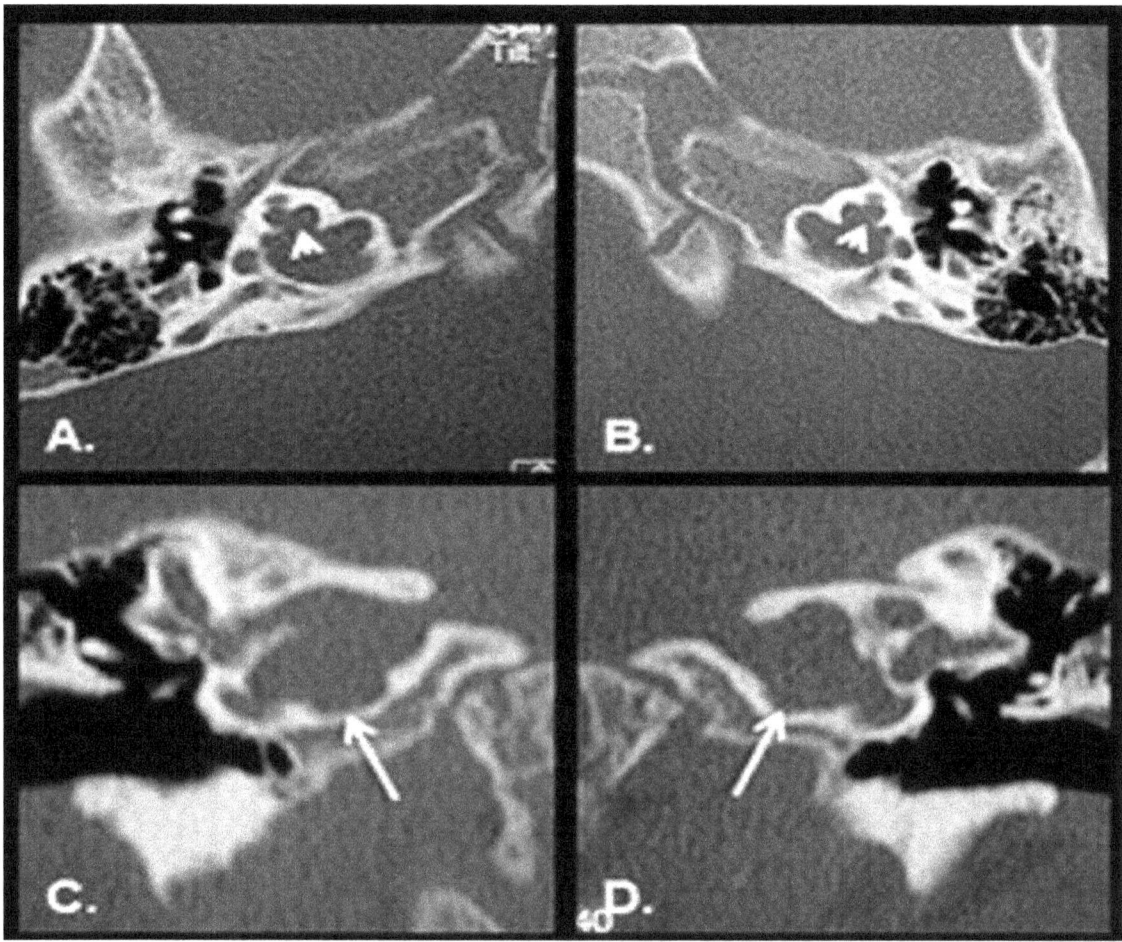

Sara J. Moren MD, Msc, Alexander W. Korutz, MD,,Achilles G. Karagranis DO,Courtney CJ Voelker, MD, PhD, Alexander J Nemeth, MD.

Images A and B demonstrate the absent of the Cochlea and Modioli. Images C and D demonstrate the internal auditory canal communicating with the Cochlea.

Audiometric Data Review

Learn to consistently review the Audiometric Data in your selected consistent systematic pattern, so you do not miss or over interpret the data. Like all other medical data (i.e.: labs and radiographs) you must compare and review all the data and compare them with the patients presenting symptoms. This consistency will reduce inappropriate additional studies to your patients and lead you to an appropriate course of medical management to your already anxious patient. If you have concerns or thoughts or question on the audiometric data you can always consult with your Audiologist.

References

David Jay Steele; Jeffrey Susman; Fredrick A. McCurdy (2003). "Student guide to primary care: making the most of your early clinical experience." Elsevier Health Sciences. pp. 370–. ISBN 978-1-56053-545-4. Retrieved 27 June 2011.

Hall III, J. W. (2000). *Handbook of Otoacoustic Emissions*, Singular Publishing Group, San Diego, CA.

Hall III, J. W.. (2014). *Introduction to Audiology Today*. Boston: Pearson Education, Inc.

Hawke, M. & McCombe, A. (1995). *Disease of the Ear: A Pocket Atlas*, Manticore Communications Inc.

Kramer, S (2014). *Audiology Science to Practice*. San Diego: Plural Publishing, Inc.

Martin, F. & Clark, J (2015). *Introduction to Audiology*. Boston: Pearson Education, Inc.

Merchant, M & Rosowski, J. (2008). "Conductive Hearing Loss Caused by Third Window Lesions of the Inner Ear." *Otol Neurotol*. 2008; 29: 282-289.

Roeser, R.J., Valente, M., Hosford-Dunn, H. (2000) *Audiology Diagnosis*. Thieme, New York. http://www.ncbi.nlm.nih.gov